ORTHOPEDIC CLINICS OF NORTH AMERICA

www.orthopedic.theclinics.com

Perioperative Pain Management

October 2017 • Volume 48 • Number 4

ELSEVIER

1600 John F. Kennedy Boulevard • Suite 1800 • Philadelphia, Pennsylvania, 19103-2899.

http://www.orthopedic.theclinics.com

ORTHOPEDIC CLINICS OF NORTH AMERICA Volume 48, Number 4
October 2017 ISSN 0030-5898, ISBN-13: 978-0-323-54674-4

Editor: Lauren Boyle
Developmental Editor: Kristen Helm

Orthopedic Clinics of North America (ISSN 0030-5898) is published quarterly by Elsevier Inc., 360 Park Avenue South, New York, NY 10010-1710. Months of issue are January, April, July, and October. Business and Editorial Offices: 1600 John F. Kennedy Blvd., Suite 1800, Philadelphia, PA 19103-2899. Customer Service Office: 3251 Riverport Lane, Maryland Heights, MO 63043. Periodicals postage paid at New York, NY and additional mailing offices. Subscription prices are $319.00 per year for (US individuals), $686.00 per year for (US institutions), $376.00 per year (Canadian individuals), $837.00 per year (Canadian institutions), $464.00 per year (international individuals), $837.00 per year (international institutions), $100.00 per year (US students), $220.00 per year (Canadian and international students). Foreign air speed delivery is included in all *Clinics* subscription prices. All prices are subject to change without notice. **POSTMASTER: Send change of address to** *Orthopedic Clinics of North America*, **Elsevier Health Sciences Division, Subscription Customer Service, 3251 Riverport Lane, Maryland Heights, MO 63043. Customer Service (orders, claims, online, change of address): Elsevier Health Sciences Division, Subscription Customer Service, 3251 Riverport Lane, Maryland Heights, MO 63043. Tel: 1-800-654-2452 (U.S. and Canada); 314-447-8871 (outside U.S. and Canada). Fax: 314-447-8029. E-mail:** journalscustomerservice-usa@elsevier.com **(for print support);** journalsonlinesupport-usa@elsevier.com **(for online support).**

Reprints. For copies of 100 or more, of articles in this publication, please contact the Commercial Reprints Department, Elsevier Inc., 360 Park Avenue South, New York, NY 10010-1710. Tel.: 212-633-3874; Fax: 212-633-3820; E-mail: reprints@elsevier.com.

Orthopedic Clinics of North America is covered in *MEDLINE/PubMed (Index Medicus), Cinahl, Excerpta Medica, and Cumulative Index to Nursing and Allied Health Literature.*

PROGRAM OBJECTIVE

Orthopedic Clinics of North America offers clinical review articles on the most cutting-edge technologies and techniques in the field, including adult reconstruction, the upper extremity, pediatrics, trauma, oncology, and sports medicine.

TARGET AUDIENCE

Practicing orthopedic surgeons, orthopedic residents, and other healthcare professionals who specialize in orthopedic technologies and techniques for adult reconstruction, the upper extremity, pediatrics, trauma, oncology, and sports medicine.

LEARNING OBJECTIVES

Upon completion of this activity, participants will be able to:

1. Review pain management considerations in foot and ankle surgeries.
2. Discuss perioperative pain management during total knee and hip arthroplasty, upper extremity surgery, and pediatric surgeries, among others.
3. Recognize methods of enhancing recovery and patient satisfaction following total knee arthroplasty.

ACCREDITATION

The Elsevier Office of Continuing Medical Education (EOCME) is accredited by the Accreditation Council for Continuing Medical Education (ACCME) to provide continuing medical education for physicians.

The EOCME designates this enduring material for a maximum of 15 *AMA PRA Category 1 Credit*(s)™. Physicians should claim only the credit commensurate with the extent of their participation in the activity.

All other healthcare professionals requesting continuing education credit for this enduring material will be issued a certificate of participation.

DISCLOSURE OF CONFLICTS OF INTEREST

The EOCME assesses conflict of interest with its instructors, faculty, planners, and other individuals who are in a position to control the content of CME activities. All relevant conflicts of interest that are identified are thoroughly vetted by EOCME for fair balance, scientific objectivity, and patient care recommendations. EOCME is committed to providing its learners with CME activities that promote improvements or quality in healthcare and not a specific proprietary business or a commercial interest.

The planning committee, staff, authors and editors listed below have identified no financial relationships or relationships to products or devices they or their spouse/life partner have with commercial interest related to the content of this CME activity:

Lauren Boyle; Blas Catalani, MD, MPH; Priscilla K. Cavanaugh, MD; Alexander C. Coleman, MD; Anjali Fortna; Tyler W. Fraser, MD; Kaela H. Frizzell, DO; Christian J. Gaffney, MD, MSc; Emmanuel Gibon, MD, PhD; Jeremy M. Gililland, MD; Marla J. Goodman, BA, MA (Int Rel); Stuart B. Goodman, MD, PhD; Kenneth W. Graf, Jr, MD; William G. Hamilton, MD; Jessica M. Kohring, MD; Rakesh P. Mashru, MD; Nathan G. Orgain, MD; Nancy L. Parks, MS; Christopher L. Peters, MD; Leslie N. Rhodes, DNP, PPCNP/BC; Christopher J. Richards, MD, MS; Matthew W. Russo, MD; Richard W. Rutherford, MD; Jeffrey R. Sawyer, MD; Benjamin W. Sheffer, MD; Jeyanthi Surendrakumar; Warren Southerland, MD; Amy Williams.

The planning committee, staff, authors and editors listed below have identified financial relationships or relationships to products or devices they or their spouse/life partner have with commercial interest related to the content of this CME activity:

Frederick M. Azar, MD is a consultant/advisor for Zimmer Biomet; 98point6 Inc; and myoscience, Inc, and has stock ownership in Campbell Clinic.

Douglas A Dennis, MD is on the speakers' bureau for, is a consultant/advisor for, has research support from, and receives royalties/patents from, DePuy Synthes, has research support from Porter Hospital, and receives royalties/patents from Wolters Kluwer.

Jesse F. Doty, MD is on the speakers' bureau for, and is a consultant/advisor for, Arthrex, Inc; Globus Medical Inc.; and Wright Medical Group N.V., and has stock ownership in Globus Medical Inc.

Martin J. Herman, MD is a consultant/advisor for, and receives royalties/patents from, DePuy Synthes and Total Joint Orthopedics, Inc.

Jason M. Jennings, MD, DPT is a consultant/advisor for DePuy Synthes and Total Joint Orthopedics, Inc.

Jerry Jones, Jr, MD is on the speakers' bureau for Halyard Health, Inc. and B. Braun Medical, Inc, is a consultant/advisor for Vocus, Inc; Halyard Health, Inc., B. Braun Medical, Inc; and Ferrosan Medical Devices, and has research support from Ferrosan Medical Devices.

Derek M. Kelly, MD receives royalties/patents from Elsevier.

Christopher E. Pelt, MD is on the speakers' bureau for Zimmer Biomet, and has research support from Zimmer Biomet and Pacira Pharmaceuticals.

UNAPPROVED/OFF-LABEL USE DISCLOSURE

The EOCME requires CME faculty to disclose to the participants:

1. When products or procedures being discussed are off-label, unlabelled, experimental, and/or investigational (not US Food and Drug Administration [FDA] approved); and

2. Any limitations on the information presented, such as data that are preliminary or that represent ongoing research, interim analyses, and/or unsupported opinions. Faculty may discuss information about pharmaceutical agents that is outside of FDA-approved labelling. This information is intended solely for CME and is not intended to promote off-label use of these medications. If you have any questions, contact the medical affairs department of the manufacturer for the most recent prescribing information.

TO ENROLL
To enroll in the *Orthopedic Clinics of North America* Continuing Medical Education program, call customer service at 1-800-654-2452 or sign up online at http://www.theclinics.com/home/cme. The CME program is available to subscribers for an additional annual fee of USD 215.

METHOD OF PARTICIPATION
In order to claim credit, participants must complete the following:
1. Complete enrolment as indicated above.
2. Read the activity.
3. Complete the CME Test and Evaluation. Participants must achieve a score of 70% on the test. All CME Tests and Evaluations must be completed online.

CME INQUIRIES/SPECIAL NEEDS
For all CME inquiries or special needs, please contact elsevierCME@elsevier.com.

EDITORIAL BOARD

CONTRIBUTORS

AUTHORS

BLAS CATALANI, MD, MPH
Clinical Instructor, Department of
Anesthesiology, The University of Tennessee
Health Science Center, Memphis, Tennessee

PRISCILLA K. CAVANAUGH, MD
Department of Orthopaedic Surgery,
Drexel University College of Medicine,
St. Christopher's Hospital for Children,
Philadelphia, Pennsylvania

ALEXANDER C. COLEMAN, MD
Staff Surgeon, Andrews Institute for
Orthopaedics & Sports Medicine,
Gulf Breeze, Florida

DOUGLAS A. DENNIS, MD
Colorado Joint Replacement, Porter Adventist
Hospital, Adjunct Professor of Bioengineering,
Department of Mechanical and Materials
Engineering, University of Denver, Assistant
Clinical Professor, Department of
Orthopaedics, University of Colorado School
of Medicine, Denver, Colorado; Adjunct
Professor, Department of Biomedical
Engineering, The University of Tennessee,
Knoxville, Tennessee

JESSE F. DOTY, MD
Assistant Professor, Department of
Orthopaedic Surgery, The University of
Tennessee, Erlanger Health System,
Chattanooga, Tennessee

TYLER W. FRASER, MD
Resident, Department of Orthopaedic
Surgery, The University of Tennessee, Erlanger
Health System, Chattanooga, Tennessee

KAELA H. FRIZZELL, DO
Department of Orthopaedic Surgery,
Philadelphia College of Osteopathic
Medicine, Philadelphia, Pennsylvania

CHRISTIAN J. GAFFNEY, MD, MSc
Department of Orthopaedics, The University
of Utah, Salt Lake City, Utah

EMMANUEL GIBON, MD, PhD
Department of Orthopaedic Surgery,
Stanford University, Stanford, California

JEREMY M. GILILLAND, MD
Assistant Professor, Department of
Orthopaedics, The University of Utah,
Salt Lake City, Utah

MARLA J. GOODMAN, BA, MA (Int Rel)
M Int Affairs, Department of Orthopaedic
Surgery, Stanford University, Stanford,
California

STUART B. GOODMAN, MD, PhD
Department of Orthopaedic Surgery,
Stanford University, Stanford, California

KENNETH W. GRAF Jr, MD
Assistant Professor of Orthopaedic Surgery,
Department of Orthopaedic Surgery, Cooper
Medical School of Rowan University, Camden,
New Jersey

WILLIAM G. HAMILTON, MD
Research Department, Anderson
Orthopaedic Research Institute,
Alexandria, Virginia

MARTIN J. HERMAN, MD
Department of Orthopaedic Surgery,
Drexel University College of Medicine,
St. Christopher's Hospital for Children,
Philadelphia, Pennsylvania

JASON M. JENNINGS, MD, DPT
Colorado Joint Replacement, Porter Adventist
Hospital, Denver, Colorado

JERRY JONES Jr, MD
Assistant Professor, Division Chief, Regional
Anesthesia and Acute Pain Medicine,
Department of Anesthesiology, The University
of Tennessee Health Science Center,
Memphis, Tennessee

DEREK M. KELLY, MD
Department of Orthopaedic Surgery and
Biomedical Engineering, Campbell Clinic,
The University of Tennessee Health Science
Center, Le Bonheur Children's Hospital,
Memphis, Tennessee

JESSICA M. KOHRING, MD
Department of Orthopaedics, The University
of Utah, Salt Lake City, Utah

RAKESH P. MASHRU, MD
Assistant Professor of Orthopaedic Surgery,
Department of Orthopaedic Surgery, Cooper
Medical School of Rowan University, Camden,
New Jersey

NATHAN G. ORGAIN, MD
Department of Anesthesiology, The University
of Utah, Salt Lake City, Utah

NANCY L. PARKS, MS
Research Department, Anderson Orthopaedic
Research Institute, Alexandria, Virginia

CHRISTOPHER E. PELT, MD
Associate Professor, Department of
Orthopaedics, The University of Utah,
Salt Lake City, Utah

CHRISTOPHER L. PETERS, MD
Professor, George S. Eccles Endowed Chair,
Department of Orthopaedics, The University
of Utah, Salt Lake City, Utah

LESLIE N. RHODES, DNP, PPCNP/BC
Department of Orthopaedic Surgery and
Biomedical Engineering, Campbell Clinic,

The University of Tennessee Health Science
Center, Le Bonheur Children's Hospital,
Memphis, Tennessee

CHRISTOPHER J. RICHARDS, MD, MS
Orthopaedic Surgery Resident, Department
of Orthopaedic Surgery, Cooper University
Health Care, Camden, New Jersey

MATTHEW W. RUSSO, MD
Research Department, Anderson Orthopaedic
Research Institute, Alexandria, Virginia

RICHARD W. RUTHERFORD, MD
Colorado Joint Replacement, Porter Adventist
Hospital, Denver, Colorado

JEFFREY R. SAWYER, MD
Department of Orthopaedic Surgery and
Biomedical Engineering, Campbell Clinic,
The University of Tennessee Health Science
Center, Le Bonheur Children's Hospital,
Memphis, Tennessee

BENJAMIN W. SHEFFER, MD
Department of Orthopaedic Surgery and
Biomedical Engineering, Campbell Clinic,
The University of Tennessee Health Science
Center, Le Bonheur Children's Hospital,
Memphis, Tennessee

WARREN SOUTHERLAND, MD
Post-Doctoral Researcher, Department
of Anesthesiology, The University of
Tennessee Health Science Center, Memphis,
Tennessee

CONTENTS

Adult Reconstruction
Patrick C. Toy

> There have been multiple successful efforts to improve and shorten the recovery period after elective total joint arthroplasty. The development of rapid recovery protocols through a multidisciplinary approach has occurred in recent years to improve patient satisfaction as well as outcomes. Bundled care payment programs and the practice of outpatient total joint arthroplasty have provided additional pressure and incentives for surgeons to provide high-quality care with low cost and complications. In this review, the evidence for modern practices is reviewed regarding patient selection and education, anesthetic techniques, perioperative pain management, intraoperative factors, blood management, and postoperative rehabilitation.

> Multimodal pain management has become the standard of care following total hip and knee replacement. The advantages include decreasing opioid consumption and its associated side effects, facilitating earlier mobilization, and faster return to function. An effective rapid recovery protocol includes the use of multiple different types of medications targeting each area of the pain pathway, preemptive analgesia, regional nerve blockade, and local infiltration analgesia.

> Total hip and knee arthroplasty is associated with significant perioperative pain, which can adversely affect recovery by increasing risk of complications, length of stay, and cost. Historically, opioids were the mainstay of perioperative pain control. However, opioids are associated with significant downsides. Preemptive use of a multimodal pain management approach has become the standard of care to manage pain after hip and knee arthroplasty. Multimodal pain management uses oral medicines, peripheral nerve blocks, intra-articular injections, and other tools to reduce the need for opioids. Use of a multimodal approach promises to decrease complications, improve outcomes, and increase patient satisfaction.

This article summarizes the current literature regarding patient satisfaction after total knee arthroplasty. In 10% to 15% of cases, the operation has not met the patients' expectations. The causes of this dissatisfaction are multifactorial and include patient-related factors, details related to the surgical procedure and prosthesis chosen, perioperative factors, and factors associated with nursing and general medical care. However, surgeons must bear the brunt of patients' dissatisfaction. This dissatisfaction erodes the doctor-patient relationship and may have implications in an emerging health care economy in which doctors and hospitals are reimbursed based on both clinical outcome and patient satisfaction.

Trauma
John C. Weinlein

The estimated rate of fracture nonunion is 5% to 10%, adding significant cost to the health care system. The cause of fracture nonunion is multifactorial, including the severity of the injury, patient factors resulting in aberrancies in the biology of fracture, and the side effects of pain control modalities. Minimizing surgeon-controlled factors causing nonunion is important to reduce the cost of health care and improve patient outcomes. Opioids, alcohol, and nonsteroidal anti-inflammatory drugs have been implicated as risk factors for fracture nonunion. Current literature was reviewed to examine the effects of opioids, alcohol, and nonsteroidal anti-inflammatory drugs on fracture union.

Postoperative pain control is a highly studied topic because of its significant effect on costs, hospital course, and, most importantly, patient satisfaction. Opioid use has been the "status quo" of postoperative pain management but prolongs hospital stays and increases complications. Optimizing acute pain management in patients with orthopedic trauma is important and can translate into significant positive physiologic and financial outcomes. Although multiple viable examples of optimizing acute pain management in the literature demonstrate outcome improvements, implementation has not been widespread. Significant outcome success will depend more on system-wide implementation than a specific regimen for postoperative pain control.

Pediatrics
Jeffrey R. Sawyer

Effective perioperative pain control in pediatric patients undergoing orthopedic surgery remains a challenge. Developing a successful pain control regimen begins preoperatively with assessment of the patient and discussion with the patient and family regarding expectations. Perioperative pain control regimens are customized based on the type of surgery, patient characteristics, and anticipated severity and duration of the postoperative pain. Recent study focuses on multimodal strategies and regional anesthesia options, allowing for decreased opioid use. This article provides an evidence-based overview of preoperative, intraoperative, and postoperative pain control for the pediatric orthopedic patient.

Pain management after spinal deformity correction surgery for scoliosis in the pediatric population can be difficult. Deformity correction with posterior spinal fusion causes significant tissue trauma. Historically, pain control has been achieved with intravenous opiates. Opiates provide excellent analgesic effect; however, they have serious consequences when used alone. In adult total joint arthroplasty, multimodal pain control has become an increasingly common method to achieve pain control without these sequelae. Recently, the same techniques have been studied in pediatric spinal deformity correction surgery. This article outlines the state of pain management in pediatric spine patients.

Upper Extremity
Benjamin M. Mauck and James H. Calandruccio

Upper extremity surgeons are currently faced with a daunting array of anesthesia techniques, ranging from traditional general anesthesia to wide-awake surgery, during which patients can watch their surgeons operate in the morning and return to work as soon as that afternoon. This range of options means that surgeons must consider patient-related factors such as disease process and relevant comorbidities, as well as surgery-related factors such as anatomic location, complexity, length of procedure, and postoperative pain expectations. In general, the least invasive technique is favored, but each patient must be considered individually to ensure the best anesthesia choice.

Foot and Ankle
Clayton C. Bettin and Benjamin J. Grear

Progress in surgical acute pain management has allowed most foot and ankle surgery to be performed in ambulatory outpatient surgical centers. Multimodal analgesia focuses on improving postoperative pain by combining pharmacologic and other modalities, addressing multiple pain mechanisms and receptor pathways while reducing adverse effects through lower doses of oral medications. Local anesthesia techniques provide excellent pain relief with few adverse events. Multimodal analgesia in foot and ankle surgery provides superior pain relief, and reduced opioid dependence and opioid-related side effects, improving patient satisfaction, safety, and timely return to function.

Postoperative pain is one of the most important factors in regard to patient outcomes. It has been linked with patient satisfaction, length of stay, and overall hospital costs. Peripheral nerve blocks have provided a safe, effective method to control early postoperative pain when symptoms are most severe. Peripheral nerve blocks, whether used intraoperatively or postoperatively, provide an alternative or adjunct to conventional pain management methods for patients who may not tolerate heavy narcotics or general anesthesia, in particular, the elderly and those with cardiopulmonary disease.

PERIOPERATIVE PAIN MANAGEMENT

PREFACE

Perioperative Pain Management

Patient satisfaction and outcomes are increasingly influencing reimbursement, and multiple studies have shown a direct correlation between increased pain and decreased patient satisfaction. The current focus on opioid overuse has made perioperative pain management a challenge. This issue of *Orthopedic Clinics of North America* highlights some of those difficulties and provides discussions of alternate pain management strategies in orthopedic patients.

With an aging population, total joint arthroplasties (TJA) are common procedures to combat end-stage joint degeneration for which conservative measures have failed. Rutherford, Jennings, and Dennis review the evidence for modern practices regarding patient selection and education, anesthetic techniques, perioperative pain management, intraoperative factors, blood management, and postoperative rehabilitation. The importance of pain management in the rapid recovery of TJA patients is highlighted by Russo, Parks, and Hamilton, with a discussion of rapid recovery protocols. Gaffney, Pelt, Gililland, and Peters present a multimodal pain management approach to avoid adverse effects of opioids while improving patient satisfaction. Although innovative surgical and pain management techniques have improved the outcomes of total knee arthroplasty, 10% to 15% of patients are dissatisfied with their results. Gibon, Marla Goodman, and Stuart Goodman present an in-depth discussion of how the multifactorial causes of patient dissatisfaction, including pain, can be addressed.

Pain control is especially important in orthopedic trauma patients, in whom opioids have traditionally been the most common choice. As pointed out by Richards, Graf, and Mashru, however, side effects of opioids and nonsteroidal anti-inflammatory medications used for pain control may impede fracture healing. Jones, Southerland, and Catalani describe methods for optimizing acute pain management in orthopedic trauma patients.

Two articles by pediatric orthopedic surgeons, one by Frizzell, Cavanaugh, and Herman and the other by Sheffer, Kelly, Sawyer, and Rhodes, discuss the challenging issue of pain control in pediatric patients, including multimodal approaches, accelerated postoperative pathways, and regimens customized according to patient and surgery characteristics that are unique to these young patients.

Because many hand and foot and ankle surgeries are done as outpatient procedures, local and regional anesthesia techniques are commonly used. Authors Coleman; Kohring and Orgain; and Fraser and Doty outline anesthesia options and methods to minimize their side effects while providing excellent pain relief. Techniques such as wide-awake surgery, wound infiltration, combinations of pharmacologic and other modalities that target multiple pain mechanisms and receptor pathways can reduce dependence on opioids.

We hope the information provided in this issue will be helpful to you in developing perioperative pain management protocols for your patients.

Frederick M. Azar, MD
Campbell Clinic, Inc
University of Tennessee-Campbell Clinic
Department of Orthopaedic Surgery &
Biomedical Engineering
1211 Union Avenue, Suite 510
Memphis, TN 38104, USA

E-mail address:
fazar@campbellclinic.com

Orthop Clin N Am 48 (2017) xiii
http://dx.doi.org/10.1016/j.ocl.2017.07.001
0030-5898/17/© 2017 Published by Elsevier Inc.

Adult Reconstruction

Enhancing Recovery After Total Knee Arthroplasty

Richard W. Rutherford, MD[a],*, Jason M. Jennings, MD, DPT[a],
Douglas A. Dennis, MD[a,b,c,d]

KEYWORDS

- Rapid recovery • Total knee arthroplasty (TKA) • Rehabilitation protocol

KEY POINTS

- Efforts to identify and correct modifiable risk factors should be undertaken before elective total knee arthroplasty (TKA).
- There is adequate evidence to support the use of multimodal pain management protocols in TKA, although debate exists over the optimal regimen.
- The advent of tranexamic acid has reduced the transfusion rate and associated complications after TKA.
- There is no consensus regarding the type, appropriate frequency, duration, or intensity of physical therapy protocols after TKA.

INTRODUCTION

Rapid or enhanced protocols to improve recovery after total knee arthroplasty (TKA) have evolved in response to efforts to improve patient satisfaction, the advent of bundled care, and the increasing practice of "fast-track" and outpatient total joint arthroplasty (TJA). The increasing demand and volume of TKAs performed have created pressure from payer sources to provide high-quality outcomes at low cost. The sharing of costs with physicians and the opportunity to share cost savings have incentivized physicians to improve preoperative, intraoperative, and postoperative care strategies. Multiple specialties, including orthopedic surgeons, anesthesiologists, and physical therapists, have contributed to improving the standard of care in "fast-track" elective TKA to make it a safe and effective procedure, even when performed in the outpatient setting. Despite these efforts, there continues to be room for improvement in patient satisfaction after TKA. Although TKA is a successful operation for most patients, there is a significant portion of patients who remain unsatisfied. In a survey of 1712 TKA patients, only 89% reported willingness to undergo another TKA,[1] and overall satisfaction was a modest 81%. A multicenter study examining patient satisfaction in young patients found that newer knee designs have not resulted in improved patient satisfaction in younger patients.[2]

PATIENT OPTIMIZATION

Recognizing which patients are at risk for adverse outcomes after TKA is the first step in preventing them. Optimizing modifiable risk factors is imperative for success, and surgery may need to be delayed until many are corrected. Routine preoperative medical evaluation by primary care specialists is valuable in identification of many of these risk factors. Although the following risk factors are discussed individually, many patients will present with a combination of these medical comorbidities.

[a] Colorado Joint Replacement, Porter Adventist Hospital, 2535 S. Downing Street, Denver, CO 80210, USA; [b] Department of Biomedical Engineering, University of Tennessee, Knoxville, TN, USA; [c] Department of Mechanical and Materials Engineering, University of Denver, Denver, CO, USA; [d] Department of Orthopaedics, University of Colorado School of Medicine, Denver, CO, USA
* Corresponding author. Colorado Joint Replacement, 2535 S. Downing Street, Suite 100, Denver, CO 80210.
E-mail address: richardwrutherford@gmail.com

Orthop Clin N Am 48 (2017) 391–400
http://dx.doi.org/10.1016/j.ocl.2017.05.002
0030-5898/17/© 2017 Elsevier Inc. All rights reserved.

Psychological

Inferior outcomes have been reported with decreased mental composite scores because of conditions such as depression and anxiety.[3] These patients may benefit from additional efforts in preoperative education and in postoperative rehabilitation. Providing additional attention to these patients through more frequent postoperative phone calls and office visits to provide psychological support can be beneficial.

Obesity

Body mass index (BMI) greater than 30 is associated with increased length of stay (LOS) and increased likelihood of discharge to a rehabilitation facility.[4] In a large database study of morbidly obese patients, BMI greater than 40 was associated with an increase in complications, mortality, and resource use, but with a relatively modest effect size when controlled for comorbid conditions.[5]

Anemia

Preoperative anemia should be screened for and corrected, if possible, before elective TKA. It has been associated with increased transfusion rate, infection risk, increased LOS,[6,7] and an increased risk of mortality.[8] Perioperative allogenic transfusions have also been associated with an increased infection rate in TKA[9] in patients with increased infection risk factors such as diabetes and obesity. A multicenter study in Europe conducted in 2015 determined that strategies to identify and treat anemic patients were still underutilized.[10]

Diabetes Mellitus

Diabetic patients are at increased risk of infection after TJA, especially those with poor glycemic control. These subjects are at increased risk of surgical and medical complications and have a higher mortality risk and increased LOS.[11] The investigators recommend monitoring HgbA1c as a marker of long-term glucose control, which should ideally be less than 8.[12] Early postoperative glucose management, which was first identified as an important part of preventing infection in cardiac and general surgery,[13] is important, even in nondiabetics. Glucose should be monitored postoperatively with a goal of 110 to 140 g/dL.[14]

Tobacco Use

Smokers are at a higher risk of multiple complications after surgical procedures, including the need for mechanical ventilation, wound healing problems, infection, and cardiac complications.[15] Smoking cessation 4 to 6 weeks before operative intervention is recommended to decrease complications.[16] A 2010 Cochrane Review showed that interventions including behavioral support and nicotine replacement therapy (NRT) can be effective in reducing postoperative morbidity.[17] Obtaining a cotinine level preoperatively is one method to monitor compliance, but for patients on NRT (who would test positive for nicotine byproducts), checking an expired carbon monoxide breathing test has been described.[15]

Malnutrition

Malnutrition places patients at higher risk of wound complications, infection, and medical complications after TKA.[18] Markers indicating malnutrition are total lymphocyte count less than 1500 cells/mm^3, albumin of less than 3.5 g/dL, and transferrin levels less than 200 mg/dL.[19] As noted by Huang and colleagues,[18] obese patients are often paradoxically malnourished, and this should be addressed before elective TKA.

PREOPERATIVE EDUCATION

There are conflicting data in the literature regarding whether preoperative education is a useful intervention for TKA patients. Noble and colleagues[20] found that patient satisfaction was highly correlated with whether preoperative expectations had been met. Culliton and colleagues[21] found no difference in patient satisfaction in regard to preoperative expectations, but did find that postoperative expectations were correlated to satisfaction, and recommend continuing patient education through the postoperative period. However, in a 2014 Cochrane Review, no significant differences were demonstrated in regard to outcomes (either pain, function, health-related quality of life, or complications) when preoperative education was evaluated. It was recognized that preoperative education may be useful in certain populations; those with depression or anxiety, and to correct unrealistic expectations.[22] Given the potential benefits of preoperative education, the negligible potential for harm, low cost, and in light of the decreasing hospital LOS, the investigators think that the importance of preoperative education will increase because patients spend less time being monitored and educated in the hospital.

INTRAOPERATIVE CONSIDERATIONS
Minimally Invasive Surgery

Minimally invasive surgery (MIS) TKA techniques have been proposed to offer benefits of less blood loss, reduced pain, and faster recovery.[23]

Examples of MIS TKA exposures include the mini-subvastus, mini-medial parapatellar, mini-midvastus, and quadriceps-sparing techniques. The hypothetical benefits of MIS approaches relate primarily to preservation of quadriceps function.[24,25] MIS techniques require specialized instrumentation to avoid component malposition, which was a reported complication early in the development of these techniques.[26] Although there can be an early benefit in mobility, 2- and 6-year outcomes with MIS and standard TKA approaches were no different in a recent study by Unwin and colleagues.[27] A prospective trial of 134 patients randomized to standard versus MIS TKA (using midvastus approach) found no difference in radiographic alignment, function, or range of motion at 1 year, although MIS TKA subjects experienced slightly less blood loss and slightly more operative time.[28]

Tourniquet Use

Intraoperative tourniquet use is recognized to be a cause of postoperative pain and was recently demonstrated to adversely affect quadriceps strength for up to 3 months postoperatively.[29] Although increased intraoperative blood loss without tourniquet was observed by Dennis and colleagues[29] in a randomized trial of 56 bilateral TKA, the total (intraoperative and postoperative) blood loss was not statistically different. Use of a tourniquet may simply delay intraoperative blood loss until after surgery, which may, in fact, be exacerbated by a paradoxic increase in bleeding due to reactive hyperemia.

Blood Management

Reducing intraoperative and postoperative blood loss can enable better mobilization and help to avoid complications such as fluid overload, increased infection rate, and increased LOS.[9,30] Transfusion rates (and associated complications) have been significantly reduced by the adoption of tranexamic acid (TXA). The most effective dosing strategy for TXA is debated, but oral, intravenous, and intraarticular dosing regimens have been shown to be effective and safe in reducing blood loss and transfusion rate in the perioperative period.[31–33] The use of fibrin sealants have been shown to reduce blood loss, but are not as cost-effective as TXA.[30]

Drain Use

Routine use of a drain, although commonly thought to reduce the incidence of hemarthrosis and facilitate mobilization, has been shown to increase blood loss.[34] In small randomized prospective studies, use of a drain has been shown to increase postoperative blood loss and has not been shown to affect short-term outcomes.[34,35] A meta-analysis involving 1361 TKAs conducted by Zhang and colleagues[36] found no difference in range of motion, quadriceps strength, or outcomes with or without the use of a drain.

PERIOPERATIVE PAIN AND FLUID MANAGEMENT

Anesthetic Methods

The objectives of most rapid recovery protocols in TKA are to provide pain relief and avoid complications, especially postoperative nausea, oversedation, and prolonged motor blockade. Neuraxial anesthesia appears to be safer and more effective than general anesthesia in TJA. In a study comparing use of neuraxial and general anesthesia in 500,000 TJAs, decreases in 30-day mortality, LOS, and cost were found when neuraxial anesthesia was used.[37] Regional anesthesia has been advocated in recent years as a method to enhance postoperative pain control. Femoral and sciatic nerve blocks have both been used but are associated with prolonged motor blockade, which interferes with early mobilization and may place patients at a risk for falls.[38] Adductor canal blocks (ACB) and periarticular injections (PAI) are recent advancements that provide equivalent pain control when compared with femoral nerve blocks, with preservation of motor function.[39,40] The use of intraoperative PAI is supported by multiple randomized controlled trials.[41–44] The authors' preferred technique is to inject multiple areas of the knee with a 22-gauge needle with small (1–2 mL) quantities, with attention to the posterior capsule, periosteum surrounding the areas of bone resection, and fat pad. It remains to be determined whether ACB, PAI, or a combination of the 2 in conjunction with spinal anesthesia provide the most optimal pain control after TKA.

Analgesia

Multimodal pain management strategies have evolved to improve patient satisfaction, improve early mobilization, and reduce complications associated with opioid monotherapy.[45,46] Opioids, which have been a mainstay of surgical pain management, have multiple adverse drug effects and have been shown to be associated with increased LOS and costs across surgical subspecialties.[47] Undertreating pain with opioid monotherapy to avoid adverse effects can lead to uncontrolled pain and slower patient mobilization. Properly addressing postoperative pain with a multimodal regimen is of the utmost importance so that participation in therapy and early discharge are possible. A typical regimen involves acetaminophen, nonsteroidal anti-inflammatory agents, opioid analgesic, with or without gabapentin or gabapentinoid medication. The use of preemptive analgesia, or medication administered before tissue injury, can dampen the inflammatory cascade in response to surgery as well as lessening pain due to neuronal hyperexcitability.[48,49] This multimodal regimen is most effective when continued postoperatively because of the prolonged transmission of stimuli from afferent pain receptors. Antiemetic medications with adjuvant short-acting corticosteroids are also useful in reducing perioperative nausea and vomiting. The use of corticosteroids in the perioperative period likely has a synergist effect with regards to decreasing both inflammation and pain.[50]

REHABILITATION

There is currently no clear consensus regarding the frequency, duration, or intensity of physical therapy protocols for TKA patients. Historical rehabilitation protocols involved an early long period of immobilization followed by delayed initiation of therapy. Early in this decade, accelerated protocols were developed that focused on early mobilization using specialized care teams. These protocols were found to reduce hospital stay and cost.[51] There is a need to establish clear targets for rehabilitation based on functional testing. The authors' current practice is typically a regimen of 2 to 3 outpatient physical therapy visits per week for 4 to 6 weeks postoperatively. The patient is educated not to depend on the therapist and to perform their regimen 3 times per day independently. Outpatient physical therapy, in contrast to home physical therapy visits, is preferred to encourage

additional patient mobility and provide better access to specialized equipment.

Preoperative Rehabilitation

Preoperative physical therapy or "prehab" has been shown to have modest effects on pain in the first 4 weeks with modest improvements in functional scores, with no difference in hospital LOS, cost, or quality of life. These effects were considered too small and fleeting to be clinically relevant in a systematic review and meta-analysis conducted by Wang and colleagues in 2016.[52] Considering the substantial reduction in hospital LOS that has occurred during this decade, the investigators favor a single preoperative physical therapy assessment, at least with patients demonstrating significant preoperative disability. This assessment can provide valuable preoperative education, determine specific home patient needs, and is often helpful in reducing preoperative patient anxiety, which can adversely affect postoperative rehabilitation.

Limb Elevation

Elevation of the lower extremity multiple times daily in the early postoperative period is imperative to lessen lower extremity edema. Increased edema adversely affects knee range of motion and speed of patient mobilization.

Cryotherapy

Cryotherapy is a useful nonpharmacologic analgesic method that is useful in the acute perioperative and postoperative setting. There are multiple devices available that have been marketed to improve pain and swelling for postsurgical patients. There has been no significant benefit in pain, swelling, or range of motion associated with these devices, when compared with traditional cold packs.[53] The authors advise caution with the use of advanced cryotherapy devices use due to the risk of thermal injury (Fig. 1). The authors' recommendation is

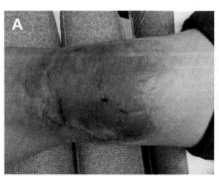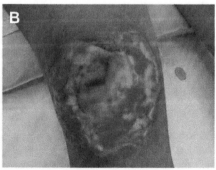

Fig. 1. (A, B) Tissue injury secondary to advanced cryotherapy devices.

traditional ice or gel packs for 20 to 30 minutes per session to minimize the risk of thermal injury.

Continuous Passive Motion
Although continuous passive motion (CPM) has been thought of as a method to improve range of motion after TKA, it has not been shown to improve range of motion, clinical outcomes, or discharge disposition.[54,55] In addition, it results in increased cost and has been associated with more persistent knee swelling.[54] Because of these factors, its use has declined in recent years. In the authors' practice, CPM is most commonly used in patients who require a closed manipulation for postoperative arthrofibrosis. These patients typically have a "defeated" attitude, and the use of CPM may provide a psychological boost to their rehabilitative efforts.

Neuromuscular Electrical Stimulation
The theory behind the use of neuromuscular electrical stimulation is that dosed electrical current used to stimulate muscle contraction may augment muscle strength. It is typically used for quadriceps strengthening, which is well recognized as part of physical rehabilitation after TKA. There are conflicting reports regarding neuromuscular stimulation, with some evidence that early intervention may be beneficial.[56] However, the current data are not sufficient to support its routine use, based on a recent Cochrane Review by Monaghan and colleagues,[57] based on the low quality of the evidence.

Balance Training
Proprioception remains altered after TKA, and some rehabilitation protocols have been developed to improve balance.[58] Although it is thought that improved balance may result in better function postoperatively, there is no clear evidence to support a specific protocol.[59–61] The authors' practice has been to incorporate weight-bearing exercises to improve muscle coordination and joint stabilization with emphasis on strength, coordination, balance, and posture.

Aquatic Therapy
Aquatic therapy, in conjunction with traditional, land-based therapy, has been shown in small trials to convey a benefit in swelling and range of motion.[62] Hydrostatic pressure from limb submersion combined with exercise can result in improvements in limb edema and may augment recovery. However, there is no high-quality evidence demonstrating a long-term benefit after TKA, and it is associated with increased costs. An additional barrier is surgeon reluctance to submerge the wound until the incision has completely healed. Further study is needed to determine specific protocols and which patients would benefit most from this as an adjunct to traditional therapy.

Pet Therapy
The use of therapy dogs has been documented in the pediatric and oncologic population and was recently studied as part of a randomized controlled trial by Harper and colleagues.[63] It was demonstrated both to improve patient satisfaction and to reduce visual analogue scale pain scores in a study of 72 Total Hip Arthroplasty (THA) and Total Knee Arthroplasty (TKA) patients. This small study suggests it may be beneficial as part of a postoperative rehabilitation program, especially in patients with anxiety, pain catastrophizers, and patients with poor coping skills. It has also been suggested that incorporating a pet therapy program on a hospital ward is beneficial for staff morale,[64] which may also contribute to higher patient satisfaction.

Lower Extremity Bracing
Static and dynamic bracing can be indicated in patients with a postoperative contracture. The 2 basic types of braces are load control, which apply a constant force across the joint, and dynamic control braces, which apply a specific amount of deformation across the knee joint.[65] There are small studies reporting effectiveness of both load control and dynamic control bracing for stiffness after TKA.[66–70] The senior author favors the use of a knee immobilizer at night for the first 3 to 4 weeks to lessen the risk of developing a flexion contracture. Dynamic extension bracing is reserved for severe cases of postoperative contracture in the authors' practice. Close communication with the physical therapist is emphasized for patients having difficulty regaining range of motion in the acute postoperative period.

Discharge Destination
Discharge destination has been shown to be an independent risk factor for adverse events and unplanned readmission.[71] The authors' practice is to discuss and plan discharge destination in advance, with strong encouragement for the patient to return home directly upon hospital discharge. There is also a significant increased cost to consider, because it has been shown that after discharge care accounts for 36% of payments for the total episode of care surrounding TJA.[72] Because of the advent of episode-of-care or bundled payments, close attention should be paid to determine whether discharge

to post–acute rehabilitation facilities is merited in light of the increased costs as well as higher comorbidity adjusted complication and readmission rates. Use of clinical care coordinators ("nurse navigators") who preoperatively assess individual patient needs, provide useful information regarding discharge destination, and monitor patients postoperatively are valuable to expedite patient rehabilitation and lessen rates of hospital readmission. They also follow patients requiring discharge to post–acute facilities to assure progress is monitored and that their LOS is kept to a minimum.

Alternative Therapy Regimens

Alternative therapy programs such as a monitored home exercise program and tele-rehabilitation have been shown to be noninferior

Table 1 Recommendations for enhanced recovery after total knee arthroplasty	
Patient optimization	
Psychological	Provide additional educational resources and support to patients with depression and anxiety
Anemia	Screen for preoperative anemia and correct before elective TKA, if possible
Diabetes	Monitor HgA1c with a goal of <8; perioperative blood glucose should ideally be kept between 110 and 140 g/dL
Tobacco use	Smoking cessation 4–6 wk before surgery with behavioral support
Malnutrition	Correct malnutrition before surgery; markers indicating malnutrition are total lymphocyte count (TLL) <1500 cells/mm^3, albumin <3.5 g/dL, and transferrin <200 mg/dL
Preoperative education	
Patient expectations	Managing patient expectations with preoperative and postoperative education has potential benefits with conflicting data in the literature
Intraoperative factors	
Tourniquet use	The authors recommend limiting tourniquet use to decrease quadriceps inhibition after TKA
Blood management	Use of TXA (either intravenous, topical, or oral) reduces blood loss and transfusions after TKA
Perioperative factors	
Anesthetic methods	Neuraxial anesthesia appears to be safer and more effective than general anesthesia in TKA
Regional and local anesthesia	Motor function–sparing adjuvant methods such as ACBs and PAIs can enhance perioperative pain control
Analgesia	Multimodal pain protocols incorporating acetaminophen, nonsteroidal anti-inflammatory drugs, gapapentinoids, short-acting corticosteroids with supplemental opioids rather than opioid monotherapy are recommended
Rehabilitation	
Physical therapy (PT)	Although there is no consensus on length, duration, or intensity of PT after TKA, the authors' practice is 2–3 outpatient visits per week for 4–6 wk
Preoperative rehabilitation	The authors favor a single preoperative PT visit, especially in those with significant preoperative disability
Cryotherapy	Traditional ice or gel packs for 20–30 min per session are recommended over cryotherapy devices due to the cost and risk of thermal injury
CPM	Use of CPM is reserved for patients who have had a closed manipulation and is not used after primary TKA
Bracing	Dynamic extension bracing is reserved for severe cases of postoperative contracture
Discharge disposition	Use of clinical care coordinators and discussing disposition in advance of surgery are recommended with strong encouragement for discharge to home

to traditional outpatient physical therapy protocols after TKA.[73,74] These programs may be used as a substitute or as an adjunct to face to face outpatient physical therapy, and if incorporated, would be expected to be associated with decreased cost. Further studies to identify which patients would benefit most from face-to-face therapy versus remote or self-directed protocols are needed.

Patient Encouragement

Recovering from a TKA is a challenging event for most patients receiving this procedure. Attempts to motivate and frequently encourage the patient, particularly by the operating surgeon, can be very helpful in facilitating patient recovery.

SUMMARY/KEY POINTS

There is good evidence to support the use of multimodal pain management protocols to reduce opioid use and enhance recovery in TJA (Table 1). Although debate exists over the optimal regimen, a combination of neuraxial anesthesia with regional blocks and local infiltration as well as a multimodal oral medication strategy that begins preoperatively and is continued postoperatively is ideal.

The advent of TXA has reduced the transfusion rate and associated complications after TKA. Oral, intravenous, and topical administration regimens have all been shown to be effective.

There is no consensus regarding the appropriate frequency, duration, or intensity of physical therapy protocols after TKA. Research is needed to determine which patients need additional resources and adjunctive treatments, and for which patients a monitored home program, or remote program, may be appropriate.

REFERENCES

1. Bourne RB, Chesworth B, Davis A, et al. Comparing patient outcomes after THA and TKA: is there a difference? Clin Orthop Relat Res 2010;468(2):542–6.
2. Nunley RM, Nam D, Berend KR, et al. New total knee arthroplasty designs: do young patients notice? Clin Orthop Relat Res 2015;473(1):101–8.
3. Franklin PD, Li W, Ayers DC. The Chitranjan Ranawat award: functional outcome after total knee replacement varies with patient attributes. Clin Orthop Relat Res 2008;466(11):2597–604.
4. Miric A, Lim M, Kahn B, et al. Perioperative morbidity following total knee arthroplasty among obese patients. J Knee Surg 2002;15(2):77–83. Available at: http://www.ncbi.nlm.nih.gov/pubmed/12013077. Accessed February 26, 2017.
5. D'Apuzzo MR, Novicoff WM, Browne JA. The John Insall Award: morbid obesity independently impacts complications, mortality, and resource use after TKA. Clin Orthop Relat Res 2015; 473(1):57–63.
6. Kotze A, Carter LA, Scally AJ. Effect of a patient blood management programme on preoperative anaemia, transfusion rate, and outcome after primary hip or knee arthroplasty: a quality improvement cycle. Br J Anaesth 2012;108(6):943–52.
7. Greenky M, Gandhi K, Pulido L, et al. Preoperative anemia in total joint arthroplasty: is it associated with periprosthetic joint infection? Clin Orthop Relat Res 2012;470(10):2695–701.
8. Spahn DR. Anemia and patient blood management in hip and knee surgery: a systematic review of the literature. Anesthesiology 2010;113(2):482–95.
9. Newman ET, Watters TS, Lewis JS, et al. Impact of perioperative allogeneic and autologous blood transfusion on acute wound infection following total knee and total hip arthroplasty. J Bone Joint Surg Am 2014;96(4):279–84.
10. Lasocki S, Krauspe R, von Heymann C, et al. PREPARE: the prevalence of perioperative anaemia and need for patient blood management in elective orthopaedic surgery: a multicentre, observational study. Eur J Anaesthesiol 2015;32(3):160–7.
11. Marchant MH, Viens NA, Cook C, et al. The impact of glycemic control and diabetes mellitus on perioperative outcomes after total joint arthroplasty. J Bone Joint Surg Am 2009;91(7):1621–9.
12. Cancienne JM, Werner BC, Browne JA. Is there an association between hemoglobin a1c and deep postoperative infection after TKA? Clin Orthop Relat Res 2017;475:1–8.
13. Gelijns AC, Moskowitz AJ, Acker MA, et al. Management practices and major infections after cardiac surgery. J Am Coll Cardiol 2014;64(4):372–81.
14. Mraovic B, Suh D, Jacovides C, et al. Perioperative hyperglycemia and postoperative infection after lower limb arthroplasty. J Diabetes Sci Technol 2011;5(2):412–8.
15. Akhavan S, Nguyen L-C, Chan V, et al. Impact of smoking cessation counseling prior to total joint arthroplasty. Orthopedics 2016;1–6. http://dx.doi.org/10.3928/01477447-20161219-02.
16. Lindström D, Azodi OS, Wladis A, et al. Effects of a perioperative smoking cessation intervention on postoperative complications. Ann Surg 2008; 248(5):739–45.
17. Thomsen T, Villebro N, Møller AM. Interventions for preoperative smoking cessation. In: Thomsen T, editor. Cochrane database of systematic reviews. Chichester (United Kingdom): John Wiley & Sons, Ltd; 2014:CD002294.

18. Huang R, Greenky M, Kerr GJ, et al. The effect of malnutrition on patients undergoing elective joint arthroplasty. J Arthroplasty 2013;28(8 SUPPL):21–4.

19. Greene KA, Wilde AH, Stulberg BN. Preoperative nutritional status of total joint patients. Relationship to postoperative wound complications. J Arthroplasty 1991;6(4):321–5. Available at: http://www.ncbi.nlm.nih.gov/pubmed/1770368. Accessed March 5, 2017.

20. Noble PC, Conditt MA, Cook KF, et al. The John Insall Award: patient expectations affect satisfaction with total knee arthroplasty. Clin Orthop Relat Res 2006;452:35–43.

21. Culliton SE, Bryant DM, Overend TJ, et al. The relationship between expectations and satisfaction in patients undergoing primary total knee arthroplasty. J Arthroplasty 2012;27(3):490–2.

22. McDonald S, Page MJ, Beringer K, et al. Preoperative education for hip or knee replacement. Cochrane Database Syst Rev 2014;(5):CD003526.

23. Tria AJ, Scuderi GR. Minimally invasive knee arthroplasty: an overview. World J Orthop 2015;6(10):804.

24. Cheng T, Liu T, Zhang G, et al. Does minimally invasive surgery improve short-term recovery in total knee arthroplasty? Clin Orthop Relat Res 2010;468(6):1635–48.

25. Alcelik I, Sukeik M, Pollock R, et al. Comparison of the minimally invasive and standard medial parapatellar approaches for primary total knee arthroplasty. Knee Surg Sports Traumatol Arthrosc 2012;20(12):2502–12.

26. Dalury DF, Dennis DA. Mini-incision total knee arthroplasty can increase risk of component malalignment. Clin Orthop Relat Res 2005;440:77–81. Available at: http://www.ncbi.nlm.nih.gov/pubmed/16239787. Accessed March 5, 2017.

27. Unwin O, Hassaballa M, Murray J, et al. Minimally invasive surgery (MIS) for total knee replacement; medium term results with minimum five year follow-up. Knee 2017;24(2):454–9.

28. Wülker N, Lambermont JP, Sacchetti L, et al. A prospective randomized study of minimally invasive total knee arthroplasty compared with conventional surgery. J Bone Joint Surg Am 2010;92(7):1584–90.

29. Dennis DA, Kittelson AJ, Yang CC, et al. Does tourniquet use in TKA affect recovery of lower extremity strength and function? a randomized trial. Clin Orthop Relat Res 2016;474(1):69–77.

30. Su EP, Su S. Strategies for reducing peri-operative blood loss in total knee arthroplasty. Bone Joint J 2016;98B(1 Supple A):153–6.

31. Nielsen CS, Jans Ø, Ørsnes T, et al. Combined intra-articular and intravenous tranexamic acid reduces blood loss in total knee arthroplasty: a randomized, double-blind, placebo-controlled trial. J Bone Joint Surg Am 2016;98(10):835–41.

32. Moskal JT, Capps SG. Meta-analysis of intravenous tranexamic acid in primary total hip arthroplasty. Orthopedics 2016;39(5):1–10.

33. Hourlier H, Reina N, Fennema P. Single dose intravenous tranexamic acid as effective as continuous infusion in primary total knee arthroplasty: a randomised clinical trial. Arch Orthop Trauma Surg 2015;135(4):465–71.

34. Li C, Nijat A, Askar M. No clear advantage to use of wound drains after unilateral total knee arthroplasty: a prospective randomized, controlled trial. J Arthroplasty 2011;26(4):519–22.

35. Omonbude D, El Masry MA, O'Connor PJ, et al. Measurement of joint effusion and haematoma formation by ultrasound in assessing the effectiveness of drains after total knee replacement. Bone Joint J 2009;92B(1).

36. Zhang Q, Guo W, Zhang Q, et al. Comparison between closed suction drainage and nondrainage in total knee arthroplasty. J Arthroplasty 2011;26(8):1265–72.

37. Memtsoudis SG, Sun X, Chiu Y-L, et al. Perioperative comparative effectiveness of anesthetic technique in orthopedic patients. Anesthesiology 2013;118(5):1046–58.

38. Kandasami M, Kinninmonth AW, Sarungi M, et al. Femoral nerve block for total knee replacement - a word of caution. Knee 2009;16(2):98–100.

39. Chun CH, Kim JW, Kim SH, et al. Clinical and radiological results of femoral head structural allograft for severe bone defects in revision TKA–a minimum 8-year follow-up. Knee 2014;21(2):420–3.

40. Spangehl MJ, Clarke HD, Hentz JG, et al. The Chitranjan Ranawat Award: periarticular injections and femoral & sciatic blocks provide similar pain relief after TKA: a randomized clinical trial. Clin Orthop Relat Res 2015;473(1):45–53.

41. Essving P, Axelsson K, Kjellberg J, et al. Reduced morphine consumption and pain intensity with local infiltration analgesia (LIA) following total knee arthroplasty. Acta Orthop 2010;81(3):354–60.

42. Fu P, Wu Y, Wu H, et al. Efficacy of intra-articular cocktail analgesic injection in total knee arthroplasty — a randomized controlled trial. Knee 2009;16(4):280–4.

43. Koh IJ, Kang YG, Chang CB, et al. Does periarticular injection have additional pain relieving effects during contemporary multimodal pain control protocols for TKA?: a randomised, controlled study. Knee 2012;19(4):253–9.

44. Ng F-Y, Ng JK-F, Chiu K-Y, et al. Multimodal periarticular injection vs continuous femoral nerve block after total knee arthroplasty: a prospective, crossover, randomized clinical trial. J Arthroplasty 2012;27(6):1234–8.

45. Lavie LG, Fox MP, Dasa V. Overview of total knee arthroplasty and modern pain control strategies. Curr Pain Headache Rep 2016;20(11):1–5.

46. Ranawat AS, Ranawat CS, Mehta A, et al. Pain management and accelerated rehabilitation for total hip and total knee arthroplasty. J Arthroplasty 2007;22(7 Suppl 3):12–5.

47. Oderda GM, Evans RS, Lloyd J, et al. Cost of opioid-related adverse drug events in surgical patients. J Pain Symptom Manage 2003;25(3):276–83.

48. Easley ME, Cushner FD, Scott WN. Insall & Scott surgery of the knee. Surg Knee 2001;473–520. http://dx.doi.org/10.1016/B978-1-4377-1503-3.00078-0.

49. Wall PD. The prevention of postoperative pain. Pain 1988;33(3):289–90. Available at: http://www.ncbi.nlm.nih.gov/pubmed/3419835. Accessed March 3, 2017.

50. Backes JR, Bentley JC, Politi JR, et al. Dexamethasone reduces length of hospitalization and improves postoperative pain and nausea after total joint arthroplasty. J Arthroplasty 2013;28(8):11–7.

51. Larsen K, Hansen TB, Thomsen PB, et al. Cost-effectiveness of accelerated perioperative care and rehabilitation after total hip and knee arthroplasty. J Bone Joint Surg Am 2009;91(4):761–72.

52. Wang L, Lee M, Zhang Z, et al. Does preoperative rehabilitation for patients planning to undergo joint replacement surgery improve outcomes? A systematic review and meta-analysis of randomised controlled trials. BMJ Open 2016;6(2):e009857.

53. Thienpont E. Does advanced cryotherapy reduce pain and narcotic consumption after knee arthroplasty? Clin Orthop Relat Res 2014;472(11):3417–23.

54. Maniar RN, Baviskar JV, Singhi T, et al. To use or not to use continuous passive motion post–total knee arthroplasty. J Arthroplasty 2012;27(2):193–200.e1.

55. Pope RO, Corcoran S, McCaul K, et al. Continuous passive motion after primary total knee arthroplasty. Does it offer any benefits? J Bone Joint Surg Br 1997;79(6):914–7.

56. Stevens-Lapsley JE, Balter JEJ, Wolfe P, et al. Early neuromuscular electrical stimulation to improve quadriceps muscle strength after total knee arthroplasty: a randomized controlled trial. Phys Ther 2012;92(2):1–17.

57. Monaghan B, Caulfield B, O'Mathúna DP. Surface neuromuscular electrical stimulation for quadriceps strengthening pre and post total knee replacement (Review). Cochrane Database Syst Rev 2010;(1). CD007177. Available at: www.cochranelibrary.com.

58. Moutzouri M, Gleeson N, Billis E, et al. The effect of total knee arthroplasty on patients' balance and incidence of falls: a systematic review. Knee Surg Sports Traumatol Arthrosc 2016. http://dx.doi.org/10.1007/s00167-016-4355-z.

59. Piva SRS, Gil ABA, Almeida GG, et al. A balance exercise program appears to improve function for patients with total knee arthroplasty: a randomized clinical trial. Phys Ther 2010;90(6):880–94.

60. Fung V, Ho A, Shaffer J, et al. Use of Nintendo Wii Fit™ in the rehabilitation of outpatients following total knee replacement: a preliminary randomised controlled trial. Physiotherapy 2012;98(3):183–8.

61. Gstoettner M, Raschner C, Dirnberger E, et al. Preoperative proprioceptive training in patients with total knee arthroplasty. Knee 2011;18(4):265–70.

62. Gibson AJ, Shields N. Effects of aquatic therapy and land-based therapy versus land-based therapy alone on range of motion edema and function after hip or knee replacement: a systematic review and meta-analysis. Physiother Can 2015;67(2):133–41.

63. Harper CM, Dong Y, Thornhill TS, et al. Can therapy dogs improve pain and satisfaction after total joint arthroplasty? a randomized controlled trial. Clin Orthop Relat Res 2015;473(1):372–9.

64. Chinner TL, Dalziel FR. An exploratory study on the viability and efficacy of a pet-facilitated therapy project within a hospice. J Palliat Care 1991;7(4):13–20. Available at: http://www.ncbi.nlm.nih.gov/pubmed/1783956. Accessed March 27, 2017.

65. McElroy MJ, Johnson AJ, Zywiel MG. Devices for the prevention and treatment of knee stiffness after total knee arthroplasty. Expert Rev Med Devices 2011;8(1):57–65.

66. Seyler TM, Marker DR, Bhave A, et al. Functional problems and arthrofibrosis following total knee arthroplasty. J Bone Joint Surg 2007;89(suppl_3):59.

67. Bonutti PM, McGrath MS, Ulrich SD, et al. Static progressive stretch for the treatment of knee stiffness. Knee 2008;15(4):272–6.

68. Bonutti PM, Marulanda GA, McGrath MS, et al. Static progressive stretch improves range of motion in arthrofibrosis following total knee arthroplasty. Knee Surg Sports Traumatol Arthrosc 2010;18(2):194–9.

69. Steffen TM, Mollinger LA. Low-load, prolonged stretch in the treatment of knee flexion contractures in nursing home residents. Phys Ther 1995;75(10):886–95 [discussion: 895–7]. Available at: http://www.ncbi.nlm.nih.gov/pubmed/7568388. Accessed March 27, 2017.

70. McGrath MS, Mont MA, Siddiqui JA, et al. Evaluation of a custom device for the treatment of flexion contractures after total knee arthroplasty. Clin Orthop Relat Res 2009;467(6):1485–92.

71. Keswani A, Tasi MC, Fields A, et al. Discharge destination after total joint arthroplasty: an analysis of postdischarge outcomes, placement risk factors, and recent trends. J Arthroplasty 2016;31(6):1155–62.

72. Bozic KJ, Ward L, Vail TP, et al. Bundled payments in total joint arthroplasty: targeting opportunities for quality improvement and cost reduction. Clin Orthop Relat Res 2014;472(1):188–93.

73. Han ASY, Nairn L, Harmer AR, et al. Early rehabilitation after total knee replacement surgery: a multicenter, noninferiority, randomized clinical trial comparing a home exercise program with usual outpatient care. Arthritis Care Res (Hoboken) 2015;67(2):196–202.

74. Moffet H, Tousignant M, Nadeau S, et al. In-home telerehabilitation compared with face-to-face rehabilitation after total knee arthroplasty: a noninferiority randomized controlled trial. J Bone Joint Surg Am 2015; 97(14):1129–41.

Perioperative Pain Management and Anesthesia

A Critical Component to Rapid Recovery Total Joint Arthroplasty

Matthew W. Russo, MD, Nancy L. Parks, MS*,
William G. Hamilton, MD

KEYWORDS

• Pain management • Arthroplasty • Multimodal • Periarticular injection • Regional anesthesia

---

KEY POINTS

- Proactive, multimodal pain management in the setting of total joint arthroplasty allows for earlier mobilization and leads to enhanced rapid recovery and patient satisfaction.
- Minimizing opioid use is the hallmark of multimodal pain management, improving the targeting of all pain pathways while decreasing perioperative nausea and enhancing rapid participation with postoperative rehabilitation.
- Combined use of local periarticular anesthetic infiltration with avoidance of excessive soft tissue dissection and appropriate use of regional anesthesia improves patient satisfaction and pain control following total joint arthroplasty.
- Failure to control pain following total joint arthroplasty increases medical costs and risk of venous thromboembolism while prolonging overall recovery and length of stay.

INTRODUCTION

Adequate pain control is a prerequisite of rapid recovery total joint arthroplasty. Patient satisfaction is often linked to appropriate perioperative pain management. The involvement of the anesthesia team in the rapid recovery protocol is critical, with contributions to multimodal analgesia owed to enhanced regional anesthesia and neuraxial techniques. The arthroplasty surgeon and anesthesiologist should aim to capitalize on the most current techniques to achieve successful multimodal pain management.

MULTIMODAL PAIN MANAGEMENT

The philosophy of multimodal pain management in the setting of total joint replacement refers to the use of multiple types of medications delivered through many different routes with the goal of targeting all pain pathways simultaneously (Fig. 1). This strategy reduces the undesired side effects of narcotic medications including nausea, vomiting, sedation, ileus, respiratory depression, and pruritus. The result is improved patient satisfaction and earlier mobilization.

Disclosure Statement: Authors of this work participate in consulting for DePuy. The research institute where this work was compiled receives grant funding for research from Biomet and from Inova Healthcare System.
Research Department, Anderson Orthopaedic Research Institute, PO Box 7088, Alexandria, VA 22307, USA
* Corresponding author.
E-mail address: nparks@aori.org

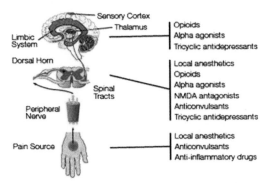

Fig. 1. Medications delivered through many different routes target multiple pain pathways. NMDA, N-methyl-D-aspartate. (©Pacira Pharmaceuticals, Inc. All Rights Reserved. Used Under License.)

PREEMPTIVE ANALGESIA

Preemptive analgesia is one of the hallmarks of multimodal pain management. By addressing pain before making the incision, the process of sensitization and production of inflammatory chemicals is prevented. With the absence of nerve fiber sensitization, the patient's pain threshold is effectively increased resulting in a decreased risk of chronic neuropathic pain and improved pain management.[1]

Treating pain before surgery allows the patient to stay ahead of the pain, which ultimately improves the efficacy of the other modes of treatment. Throughout the postoperative and rehabilitation phases, taking pain medication prophylactically keeps pain to a minimum and avoids peaks of discomfort that may interfere with recovery (Fig. 2).

MEDICATIONS

Preemptive analgesic medications are typically administered in the preoperative holding area 1 to 2 hours before the procedure but may also be initiated days before surgery. These medications typically include nonsteroidal anti-inflammatory medications (NSAIDs), cyclooxygenase (COX)-2 inhibitors, gabapentinoids, and acetaminophen (Table 1).

COX-2 inhibitors are particularly attractive for total joint replacement patients because of their reduced risk of gastric and platelet effects compared with other traditional NSAIDs. These medications have been shown to improve pain scores in total knee arthroplasty (TKA) patients with less opioid consumption and improved range of motion when analyzed in multiple randomized control trials.[2] However, in doses greater than 400 mg daily, COX-2 inhibitors increase the risk of cardiac events and should be used cautiously in patients with active cardiac disease.[3]

Glucocorticoids, specifically dexamethasone and methylprednisolone, are beneficial in the role of preemptive analgesia by decreasing the postoperative inflammatory response. These medications are often given at the time of surgery by the anesthesiologist and work together as an adjuvant treatment to prolong analgesia while reducing nausea and vomiting. Furthermore, they have been used safely without increasing wound complications with short-term use.[4]

One of the effects of preemptive analgesia is reducing narcotic consumption in the perioperative period. Although opioids still play a central

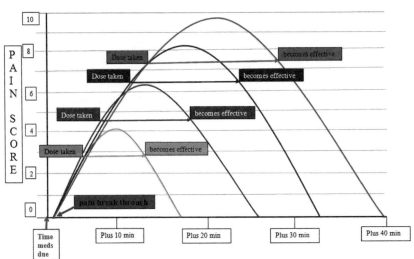

Fig. 2. To stay ahead of the pain curve, medication is best administered before high pain levels build up. (Courtesy of www.BoneSmart.org.)

Table 1
Nonopioid medications administered for preemptive analgesia

Medication	Dose, mg	Route	Preoperative, h	Postoperative
Ketorolac	15–30	Oral/intravenous	1–2	15–30 mg every 6 h
Celecoxib	400	Oral	1–2	200 mg daily
Gabapentin	300	Oral	1–2	300 mg × 1 after 24 h
Pregabalin	75	Oral	1–2	75 mg × 1 after 12 h
Acetaminophen	1000	Oral/intravenous	0–2	650 mg every 6 h

role in controlling postoperative pain, reducing them improves patient satisfaction and curtails complications related to nausea, vomiting, ileus, respiratory depression, and cognitive dysfunction, especially in the elderly patient.[5]

NEURAXIAL ANESTHESIA

One of the most important advances in rapid recovery protocol for joint replacement patients is the use of short-acting spinal/epidural anesthesia. In a study evaluating general versus neuraxial anesthesia in more than 500,000 patients undergoing TKA, general anesthesia patients had higher rates of pulmonary complications, pneumonia, infections, acute renal failure, 30-day mortality, and prolonged hospital length of stay.[6,7]

Using primarily anesthetic agents, such as lidocaine or bupivacaine, and limiting narcotic use in the spinal anesthesia has a dual benefit. It reduces opioid-related side effects, and a short-acting anesthetic allows the patient to participate in physical therapy shortly after their procedure. Lidocaine is ideal in the neuraxial anesthesia because of its much shorter duration than bupivacaine. Lidocaine typically works fast, with a short initial onset, and only lasts for 1 to 2 hours, whereas bupivacaine typically lasts 4 to 8 hours, depending on the dose. Concern about transient radiculitis, a rare side effect of

lidocaine, has caused some anesthesiologists to eschew lidocaine in favor of bupivacaine.

REGIONAL ANESTHESIA

Regional nerve blocks are another component to a successful multimodal program (Table 2).[8] The two most common regional blocks used in TKA are the femoral nerve block and the more distal adductor canal block. The femoral nerve block can result in quadriceps weakness causing falls and prolonged time to ambulation because of its mixed motor and sensory involvement.[9] The adductor canal block primarily targets sensory nerve fibers. The adductor canal block results in a sensory blockade of the anteromedial knee from the superior patella to the medial leg with minimal decrease in quadriceps strength.[10]

LOCAL INFILTRATION ANALGESIA

Although regional nerve blocks are effective for decreasing pain following TKA, they do not address many of the pain generators within the joint itself. The introduction of an anesthetic "cocktail" injection has improved pain management following total joint surgery by infusing a combination of medications directly into the soft tissues surrounding the joint space, including the posterior capsule, synovium, and periosteum. Our injection technique begins

Table 2
Anesthetic medications used for regional nerve blocks

Regional Nerve Block Medication	Lidocaine	Mepivacaine	Bupivacaine	Ropivacaine
Maximum dose, mg/kg	4.5	4.5	3	3
Dose with epinephrine, mg/kg	7	7.5	3	3
Strength, %	1–2	1.5–2	0.125–0.75	0.25–0.75
Volume, mL	10–30	10–40	10–40	15–30
Anesthesia duration, h	2–5	2–5	5–15	4–10
Duration of analgesic effect	Up to 8 h	Up to 8 h	Up to 30 h	Up to 24 h

posterior to the joint and proceeds anterior. Starting with the posterior capsule, we infuse 10 mL being careful to aspirate before injecting to ensure no vascular structure is injected. Next, 20 mL is injected into the periosteum of the femur and tibia, followed by 20 mL into the anterior femoral fat pad/synovium and extensor mechanism. The final 10 mL is infused in the subcutaneous tissues.

The role of local infiltration analgesia has continued to evolve since 2006 when the first randomized controlled trial was performed demonstrating its effectiveness.[11] Since that time, multiple studies have confirmed the efficacy of injecting a combination of a long-acting anesthetic, NSAID, steroid, and epinephrine into the soft tissues surrounding the hip or knee. Recently, multiple randomized controlled trials have been performed demonstrating

similar pain scores but improved quad strength with local infiltration analgesia compared with femoral nerve block in TKA patients.[12,13] There are a wide variety of ingredients and concentrations used, with the key ingredient of an NSAID, such as ketorolac, in the injection.[14] There is not sufficient evidence in the literature to endorse liposomal bupivacaine in the setting of total hip and knee replacement as superior to its cheaper alternatives when multimodal analgesia is performed.[15] We have found no difference in our patient population and do not currently use it at our institution. The author's preferred mixture includes

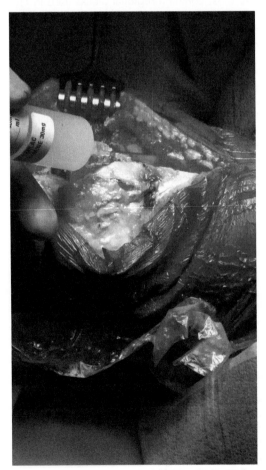

Fig. 3. Local infiltration analgesia in a total knee patient infuses a combination of medications directly into the soft tissues surrounding the joint space. Local infiltration analgesia injection of the vastus medialis oblique muscle. Just below that the synovial sleeve and femur periosteum have been injected.

Box 1
Timeline of standard multimodal pain management

1. Preoperative medications
    Tylenol, 1 g
    Oxycontin, 10 mg
    Celebrex, 400 mg
    Lyrica, 75 mg
    Scopolamine patch
2. Anesthesia: single-shot spinal
    2% Lidocaine, 75 mg
    Sufentanil, 7 μg
3. Intraoperative anesthesia
    Propofol sedation
    Zofran, 4 mg
    Dexamethasone, 4 mg
4. TKA regional block
    Adductor canal block: 0.5% ropivacaine, 25 mL
5. Local infiltration analgesia (60-mL syringe mixed with normal saline)
    0.5% ropivacaine, 30 mL
    Morphine, 10 mg
    Ketorolac, 30 mg
    Depomedrol, 40 mg
    Epinephrine, 0.5 mg
6. Postoperative medication
    Ketorolac, 30 mg once
    [a]Tylenol, 650 mg q 4
    Ultram, 50 mg q 6
    Norco, 5/325 q 4 PRN
    Celebrex, 200 mg

[a] No more than 3 g of acetaminophen in 24 hours.

0.5% ropivacaine, 30 mL; morphine, 10 mg; ketorolac, 30 mg; depomedrol, 40 mg; and epinephrine, 0.5 mg mixed in a 60-mL syringe with normal saline (Fig. 3).

Box 1 shows a standard protocol for a patient younger than 65 years old with no allergies, in overall good health, and with no comorbidities or renal disease.

SUMMARY

Adherence to a multimodal pain management protocol minimizes the undesired effects of opioid medications and allows for rapid recovery following joint replacement. Inadequate pain control following total joint replacement has the potential to create complications, readmissions, and unnecessary procedures with costly diagnostic tests and imaging.[16] A patient who is in significant pain is less likely to be satisfied with decreased mobilization and higher risk for venous thromboembolism and pulmonary complications.

REFERENCES

1. Woolf CJ, Chong MS. Preemptive analgesia: treating postoperative pain by preventing the establishment of central sensitization. Anesth Analg 1993; 77:362–79.

2. Lin J, Zhang L, Yang H. Perioperative administration of selective cyclooxygenase-2 inhibitors for postoperative pain management in patients after total knee arthroplasty. J Arthroplasty 2013; 28:207–13.e2.

3. Graham DJ. COX-2 inhibitors, other NSAIDs, and cardiovascular risk: the seduction of common sense. JAMA 2006;296:1653–6.

4. Mathiesen O, Jacobsen LS, Holm HE, et al. Pregabalin and dexamethasone for postoperative pain control: a randomized controlled study in hip arthroplasty. Br J Anaesth 2008;101:535–41.

5. Monk TG, Weldon BC, Garvan CW, et al. Predictors of cognitive dysfunction after major noncardiac surgery. Anesthesiology 2008;108:18–30.

6. Memtsoudis SG, Sun X, Chiu YL, et al. Perioperative comparative effectiveness of anesthetic technique in orthopedic patients. Anesthesiology 2013;118:1046–58.

7. Pugely AJ, Martin CT, Gao Y, et al. Differences in short-term complications between spinal and general anesthesia for primary total knee arthroplasty. J Bone Joint Surg Am 2013;95:193–9.

8. Macfarlane AJ, Prasad GA, Chan VW, et al. Does regional anesthesia improve outcome after total knee arthroplasty? Clin Orthop Relat Res 2009; 467:2379–402.

9. Sharma S, Iorio R, Specht LM, et al. Complications of femoral nerve block for total knee arthroplasty. Clin Orthop Relat Res 2010;468:135–40.

10. Moucha CS, Weiser MC, Levin EJ. Current strategies in anesthesia and analgesia for total knee arthroplasty. J Am Acad Orthop Surg 2016;24: 60–73.

11. Busch CA, Shore BJ, Bhandari R, et al. Efficacy of periarticular multimodal drug injection in total knee arthroplasty. A randomized trial. J Bone Joint Surg Am 2006;88:959–63.

12. Fan L, Yu X, Zan P, et al. Comparison of local infiltration analgesia with femoral nerve block for total knee arthroplasty: a prospective, randomized clinical trial. J Arthroplasty 2016;31:1361–5.

13. Parvataneni HK, Shah VP, Howard H, et al. Controlling pain after total hip and knee arthroplasty using a multimodal protocol with local periarticular injections: a prospective randomized study. J Arthroplasty 2007;22:33–8.

14. Kelley TC, Adams MJ, Mulliken BD, et al. Efficacy of multimodal perioperative analgesia protocol with periarticular medication injection in total knee arthroplasty: a randomized, double-blinded study. J Arthroplasty 2013;28:1274–7.

15. Hamilton TW, Athanassoglou V, Mellon S, et al. Liposomal bupivacaine infiltration at the surgical site for the management of postoperative pain. Cochrane Database Syst Rev 2017;(2):CD011419.

16. Mesko NW, Bachmann KR, Kovacevic D, et al. Thirty-day readmission following total hip and knee arthroplasty: a preliminary single institution predictive model. J Arthroplasty 2014;29:1532–8.

Perioperative Pain Management in Hip and Knee Arthroplasty

Christian J. Gaffney, MD, MSc, Christopher E. Pelt, MD,
Jeremy M. Gililland, MD, Christopher L. Peters, MD*

KEYWORDS

- Pain • Multimodal pain management • Total hip arthroplasty • Total knee arthroplasty

KEY POINTS

- Adequate pain control after hip and knee arthroplasty is essential to maximize postoperative rehabilitation, minimize complications, and ensure patient satisfaction.
- Opioid use, preoperatively and postoperatively, is associated with acute side effects, slower rehabilitation, increased complications, and the risk of tolerance and dependence.
- Multimodal analgesia is a strategy to reduce opioid consumption using various pharmacologic and interventional techniques: cryotherapy, NSAIDs, neuromodulators, peripheral nerve blocks, intra-articular injections, among others.

INTRODUCTION

Osteoarthritis (OA), also known as degenerative joint disease, affects approximately 27 million people in the United States.[1] For OA of the hip and knee, nonoperative management is directed at reducing pain and functional impairment. Conservative measures include weight loss, activity modification, physical therapy, acetaminophen, nonsteroidal anti-inflammatory drugs (NSAIDs), and intra-articular injections of glucocorticoids and hyaluronic acid. When nonoperative treatment fails, and intolerable pain and disability are present, total joint arthroplasty is a widely accepted treatment.

Total knee replacement (TKA) and total hip replacement (THA) are two of the most common surgeries performed today. The alleviation of pain, usually stemming from OA, is a primary indication for TKA and THA. Both surgeries predictably alleviate pain in most patients postoperatively. However, in the acute postoperative period, TKA and THA can cause significant pain. The fear of acute postoperative pain has been cited as a reason why patients put off arthroplasty surgery.[2] TKA, in particular, has a reputation for being an especially painful procedure from which to recover. It is not uncommon for patients to be thrilled with the results of their TKA surgery months afterward, but often state that they are unsure whether they would undergo the procedure again, now knowing how intense the immediate postoperative pain would be.

In 1995, the American Pain Society declared that pain is "the fifth vital sign." Shortly afterward, the Joint Commission on Accreditation of Healthcare Organizations said that patients should have a "right" to adequate pain management. These declarations came as evidence continued to mount demonstrating the impact of pain in patients' lives. Indeed, the orthopedic and pain literature show that if pain is not adequately controlled after TKA or THA, several detrimental pathophysiologic processes are set in motion. These processes increase the risk of

Disclosure Statement: C.E. Pelt receives institutional research support from Pacira Pharmaceuticals. The authors have nothing else to disclose related to this article.
Department of Orthopaedics, The University of Utah, 590 Wakara Way, Salt Lake City, UT 84108, USA
* Corresponding author.
E-mail address: chris.peters@hsc.utah.edu

complications and morbidity, disrupt sleep, cause cognitive dysfunction, and increase patient anxiety. Specific medical morbidities associated with inadequate pain control include venous thrombosis, coronary ischemia, myocardial infarction, and pneumonia.[3] In addition, uncontrolled pain hinders physical therapy and rehabilitation, thereby increasing the length of hospital stay and escalating the cost of care. Furthermore, the failure to control pain also leads to worse patient satisfaction with their surgery. As such, orthopedic and anesthesia providers must recognize the importance of managing pain after TKA and THA.

THE BIOLOGY AND PSYCHOLOGY OF SURGICAL PAIN

Pain is defined as "an unpleasant sensory and emotional experience associated with actual or potential tissue damage."[4] From the time the incision is made for either TKA or THA, the nociceptor pain system is activated. This includes the activation of pathways in the peripheral and the central nervous systems. Unavoidably, tissue is damaged during total joint arthroplasty. This direct damage produces a noxious stimulus that is detected by nociceptors in the peripheral nervous system. The signal is transmitted, via action potentials, to the spinal cord and then to the central nervous system. In addition to the noxious stimulus from the direct tissue damage, postoperative inflammation also leads to cell injury, and serves as a second source of pain. Furthermore, Dalury and colleagues[5] have noted that following direct tissue injury and postoperative inflammation, there is a release of inflammatory substances and cytokines including hydrogen and potassium, histamine, serotonin, prostaglandins, leukotrienes, thromboxane, and substance P.

Knowledge of the physiology of acute pain has improved greatly in recent years. Information is gathered from basic science and clinical studies from various disciplines. Although the mechanisms and physical chemistry of pain are well understood, patients have variable responses to pain.

The psychology of pain seems to be just as important as the biology, and effective pain control must take this into consideration. For example, Riddle has explored how patients' psychological status influences their perception of pain after TKA by focusing on the roles of depression, anxiety, and coping mechanisms. His group found that pain catastrophizing was a consistent predictor of poor outcome after

TKA.[6] Given there are physiologic and psychological components of pain, surgeons must consider the many options available to best manage the impact of perioperative pain and improve patient outcomes.

OPIOIDS

Opioid therapy has traditionally provided the foundation of pain control in the postoperative period for orthopedic surgery and other surgical disciplines. Oral, intravenous (IV), intramuscular, subcutaneous, transdermal, and other delivery methods are available, in a myriad of strengths and combination formulas. Some of the most commonly used opioids are morphine, hydromorphone, oxycodone, hydrocodone, and fentanyl. Morphine is one of the earliest, and still most commonly used opioids. Its use is so ubiquitous, that opioid use is often measured in terms of the equivalent morphine dose.

Opioids act by binding to opioid receptors, which are principally found in the central nervous system, the peripheral nervous system, and the gastrointestinal tract. These receptors mediate the somatic and psychoactive effects of opioids. Somatic effects include the desired pain control, and itchiness, nausea, somnolence, respiratory depression, and constipation. Psychoactive effects include euphoria in some patients. Tolerance and dependence develop with continuous use, requiring increasing doses to achieve the same effects. Withdrawal symptoms also develop if long-term use is discontinued abruptly.

The most common strategy for treating postoperative pain is to administer opioids in response to escalating pain. When managed *pro re nata* (translated as "in the circumstances"), opioid administration is often delayed by the patient waiting too long to request it and the nurse being able to provide the medicine. This process has been shown to reduce the effect of the medicine.[7] Alternatively, IV opioids are administered via a patient controlled analgesia (PCA) device that administers a dose of IV opioid when the patient pushes a button. Although appealing in that it shortens the time from pain sensation to medicine administration, adverse effects are associated with PCA use. These include sedation and somnolence, respiratory depression, nausea and vomiting, and constipation and urinary retention.[8] These side effects, coupled with the lack of evidence showing that PCA is superior to nurse-provided analgesia, has led to PCA losing popularity for pain control after arthroplasty.[9]

The efficacy of opioids in treating pain from OA has been demonstrated in studies that showed effective reduction in pain and improvements in sleep and mood. As such, opioids were increasingly used as treatment of OA-related pain in the late 1990s and early 2000s.[10] Guidelines from the American College of Rheumatology, the American Geriatrics Society, and the American Pain Society support the use of opioids for chronic OA pain. Although they are effective in alleviating pain, the previously mentioned negative side effects mean that opioids should not be the only means of treating pain after THA and TKA. Indeed, several papers have shown that opioid use actually increases complication rates after total joint arthroplasty.[11–13] That combined with the opioid epidemic should encourage surgeons to exercise caution when using opioid medications.

In addition to being aware of the side effects of opioids and cognizant of the current epidemic, the surgeon must consider each patient individually when determining a plan for perioperative pain management. This includes the patient's preoperative use of opioids. In 2016, Sing and colleagues[14] studied preoperative opioid use in patients who underwent THA or TKA for OA. The patients' home medicines before surgery were reviewed and patients were stratified according to whether they used long-acting opioids, short-acting opioids, or no opioids. The three groups were matched by age, sex, and procedure. The paper showed that the mean milligram of morphine equivalents administered in hospital was significantly higher for the opioid users (46 mg by nonusers vs 102 mg by short-acting users vs 366 mg by long-acting users). Additionally, the opioid users also reported higher visual analog pain scores throughout their hospitalization. Regarding patient outcomes, opioid users walked shorter distances on postoperative Day 1, had longer hospital stays, were more likely to be discharged to a facility instead of home, and had more complications within 90 days of surgery. They conclude that preoperative opioid use is a risk factor for slower recovery, increased cost, and increased complications after THA and TKA.

Aware of the increased risks associated with preoperative opioid use, Nguyen and colleagues[15] assessed whether weaning opioid use preoperatively would improve outcomes following THA and TKA. Their recent study retrospectively defined three cohorts of patients: (1) intervention (patients who successfully weaned their equivalent morphine dose by 50% preoperatively), (2) opioid-dependent control (patients taking opioids regularly preoperatively), and (3) an opioid naive control. The intervention group reduced their opioid use either on their own, or through guidance from their primary care doctor or a pain specialist. The three groups were matched by demographic and disease-specific variables. Compared with the opioid-dependent group, the intervention group had significantly higher increases from baseline in their postoperative physical functional scores (eg, the University of California at Los Angeles [UCLA] activity score, the Western Ontario and McMaster Universities Osteoarthritis Index [WOMAC], and the 12-Item Short Form Survey [SF-12]). The intervention group also had higher scores at final follow-up. Overall, the weaned group performed more similarly to the naive group than to their dependent matches. This study indicates that weaning preoperative opioid use can return a patient's postoperative recovery to more closely resemble an opioid-naive patient.

In summary, opioids, although effective, are associated with some adverse effects and poor outcomes. As such, multimodal options to reduce the amount of opioid medications required seem to be an effective philosophy.

MULTIMODAL PAIN MANAGEMENT

The term multimodal pain management was first introduced by Wall in 1988.[16] Wall described multimodal pain management as a strategy that incorporates various medicinal and nonmedicinal techniques of providing pain relief. The strategy targets different steps of the aforementioned pain pathways, thereby decreasing the need for opioid pain medicines postoperatively. Multimodal pain management was popularized later in a paper by Kehlet and Dahl,[17] in which they referred to it as "balanced analgesia," although this term never stuck.

When discussing multimodal pain control, Dahl and Kehlet[18] also stressed the importance of preemptive analgesia. They were pioneers in the belief that by administering medicines before surgery, one could prevent pain nociceptors from entering a state of hyperalgesia. This term refers to the sensitization of peripheral nociceptors following mechanical or thermal injury. The resultant allodynia manifests as amplified and prolonged postoperative pain, and possibly persistent, chronic pain. If the pathway toward hyperalgesia could be disrupted, this would make acute postoperative pain easier to control, with a decreased need for opioids.

Multimodal pain management includes preoperative, intraoperative, and postoperative techniques. In its broadest interpretation, multimodal management even includes preoperative patient education and discussion about pain control and expectations. Patients should have realistic expectations, goals, and education set in the preoperative period to help prepare them for their postoperative care. Preoperative education can influence a patient's perception of postoperative pain, ambulation and rehabilitation goals, and expectations for length of stay and discharge. Many institutions have created formalized preoperative patient education programs for patients undergoing joint replacement. At our institution, this program, called Joint Academy, is led by our nurses, physician assistants, physical therapists, and nurse coordinators. Furthermore, in addition to these staff members, other members of the care team provide counseling and follow several key guidelines that we believe are important for a successful preoperative education program:

- Include patients and family members in the program.
- Have representation or input from the surgical and anesthesia teams, nursing, and physical and occupational therapy.
- Describe the postoperative rehabilitation program, including goals and expectations for specific days and weeks after surgery.
- List the methods used for perioperative pain control and set reasonable expectations for postoperative pain levels.

Although the preoperative education is often provided weeks or even months before surgery, the day of surgery is another window of opportunity for intervening the patients postoperative pain experience. In preoperative holding, preemptive analgesia is often administered. Preemptive analgesia limits the sensitization of the nervous system to the painful surgical stimuli by blocking the transmission of noxious efferent information from the peripheral nervous system to the spinal cord and brain. Thus, to be effective, the medicines must be given before incision. Common agents used for preemptive analgesia include long- and short-acting opioids, acetaminophen, centrally acting synthetic analgesics, and NSAIDs. Additionally, the use of clonidine and ketamine has been reported, although they are used less frequently.[19,20]

In addition to administering pharmacologic agents, anesthesiologists can perform regional anesthetic procedures during the preoperative period to make postoperative pain easier to control and limit the actual perception of painful stimuli during and after the surgical procedure. Such procedures are integral to the practice of multimodal pain management and are discussed later.

In conjunction with the preoperative regional anesthetics described previously, intraoperative injections or periarticular infiltration (PAI) of anesthetics or medications may also be provided by the surgeon. The surgeon has multiple agents available for periarticular injection during the surgery, discussed in more detail later, which may include traditional opioids, anti-inflammatories, and local anesthetics including liposomal bupivacaine (LB).

Postoperatively, multimodal regimens include cryotherapy, pharmacologic agents, and the continued use of preoperatively placed regional anesthetics. Pharmacologic agents discussed are acetaminophen/paracetamol; NSAIDs including cyclooxygenase (COX)-2 inhibitors; centrally acting synthetic analgesics; and anticonvulsants, which have been used for treating neuropathic pain. Also, if a regional block was not used preoperatively, it is performed postoperatively if pain is uncontrolled.

CRYOTHERAPY

Cryotherapy involves the application of a bag of ice or cooled water to the skin surrounding the surgical site. Cryotherapy has long been a mainstay of postoperative pain control, and although often overlooked because of its simplicity, should be considered a component of multimodal analgesia. By lowering the temperature of the surrounding, damaged tissue, cryotherapy decreases postoperative pain in several ways, making it an intrinsically multimodal agent itself[21]: it decreases tissue metabolism and enzymatic activity (including the activity of the COX enzymes); it reduces nerve signal transduction, providing a direct analgesic effect and reducing the development of subsequent hyperalgesia; and it induces vasoconstriction and reduces extravasation of blood into surrounding tissues. This reduces blood loss and secondary inflammation.

Although most orthopedic surgeons, and the medical community overall, agree that cryotherapy is effective for pain control, the literature is equivocal. Some studies show a benefit, whereas others show little to no difference.[22,23] These studies contain small numbers of patients, are nonrandomized, and unblinded. As such, more research is needed on the benefits of cryotherapy for THA and TKA.

PARACETAMOL

Paracetamol (Tylenol) is an analgesic and antipyretic. The exact mechanism of action is not known, with early theories focusing on inhibition of COX enzymes, and contemporary research favoring a role in cannabinoid pathways. Tylenol is considered the most basic adjunct to a multimodal regimen. Caution must be used in patients with hepatic disease, because paracetamol is metabolized by the liver, and high doses can lead to hepatotoxicity and death. To decrease the incidence of hepatotoxicity, the Food and Drug Administration in 2011 asked manufacturers to discontinue any pill containing more than 325 mg of acetaminophen. Also in 2011, acetaminophen manufacturers lowered the maximum recommended daily dose from 4 g to 3 g.

In a 2008 Cochrane Review, Toms and colleagues[24] reported on the efficacy of a single dose of paracetamol (from 600 mg to 1000 mg) for treating acute postoperative pain in adults. The review evaluated 51 randomized, double-blind, placebo-controlled trials. The trials included various types of surgeries: abdominal, orthopedic, thoracic, vascular, gynecologic, and dental surgeries. In summary, they found that a single dose of acetaminophen provided effective pain relief for about half of participants experiencing moderate to severe pain after an operation. Aside from oral paracetamol, an IV option has recently been introduced. However, IV paracetamol is costly and has not been shown to provide greater pain relief in the acute postoperative setting compared with its oral counterpart in total joint arthroplasty cases.[25] Additionally, Kelly and colleagues[26] report no benefit in decreasing perioperative opioid consumption in patients who underwent TKA and received IV paracetamol versus TKA patients who did not receive IV paracetamol. Finally, a recent systematic review demonstrated no clear benefit of using IV versus oral paracetamol and recommended the use of an oral dosage for patients who are able to take oral medications in cardiology, maxillofacial, and orthopedic populations.[27]

NONSTEROIDAL ANTI-INFLAMMATORY DRUGS AND CYCLOOXYGENASE-2 INHIBITORS

Inflammation is the body's response to injury and infection, and plays an important role in postoperative pain. Although inflammation is beneficial in that it leads to the removal of offending factors and the restoration of homeostasis, the associated pain is detrimental to recovery from arthroplasty. Prostaglandins are lipid derivatives that play a key role in the inflammatory response. Derived from arachidonic acid, prostaglandins are produced by the COX enzymes, COX-1 and COX-2. Patients with higher

prostaglandin E_2 levels are slower to progress with physical therapy (eg, time to walk milestone distances, get out of bed, and climb stairs).[28]

By inhibiting the COX enzymes, NSAIDs and COX-2 inhibitors are effective for perioperative analgesia. These agents are available in various onset times, durations, routes of administration, efficacy, and side effect profiles. As such, they are a cornerstone of multimodal treatment regimens. Despite their efficacy, NSAIDs must be used with caution, because they have a significant side effect profile: gastrointestinal mucosal damage and renal dysfunction. Thus, they are contraindicated in patients with pre-existing gastrointestinal ulcers or renal impairment. Because platelet activation depends on downstream components of the prostaglandin pathway, NSAIDs also lead to increased perioperative blood loss. Many authors recommend discontinuation of NSAIDs 7 to 10 days before elective arthroplasty because studies have shown a two-fold increase in blood loss after THA.[29] Fortunately, selective COX-2 blockers have minimal gastrointestinal and hemostatic effects. Because of the lowered bleeding risk of COX-2 inhibitors, they are often coadministered with antithrombotic agents, if there is concern for thrombosis in the postoperative period.[30]

Multiple studies have demonstrated the efficacy of NSAIDs and COX-2 inhibitors in arthroplasty. Buvanendran and colleagues[31] performed a randomized, placebo-controlled, double-blind trial using the selective COX-2 inhibitor rofecoxib. The study randomized TKA patients to receive either oral rofecoxib or a placebo. The patients received their medicine before and for 2 weeks after surgery. Patients in the treatment arm had less pain, nausea, and sleep disturbance. They also consumed fewer morphine equivalents of opioids. Moreover, patients with higher plasma levels of the COX-2 inhibitor preoperatively consumed less opioids afterward. Importantly, the treatment group also demonstrated improved active and passive knee range of motion at the time of hospital discharge and 1 month after surgery. Finally, the rofecoxib group showed higher patient satisfaction at discharge and at the 2 week and 1 month follow-up visits. Of note, none of the patients had any bleeding complications.

CENTRALLY ACTING SYNTHETIC ANALGESICS

Tramadol (Ultram) is a synthetic opioid with unique properties, and thus deserves special attention because of its widespread use and increasing popularity. Tramadol is an opioid available in an oral formulation. It is unique in that it has two mechanisms. First, similar to traditional opioids like morphine and oxycodone, it binds to the μ-opioid receptor. Second, similar to some antidepressants, it also blocks the reuptake of serotonin and norepinephrine. Because of its low affinity for the mu-opioid receptor, it causes less respiratory depression, cardiac depression, dizziness, and drowsiness than traditional opioids.[32] As such, many advocate tramadol as a first-line analgesic for postoperative pain.

Aware of the adverse side effects of traditional opioids and NSAIDs, Mochizuki and colleagues[33] compared a tramadol/acetaminophen (TRAM/APAP) combination pill with NSAIDS for the treatment of perioperative pain after TKA. The TRAM/APAP studied contained 37.5 mg tramadol and 325 mg acetaminophen. The NSAIDs studied were lornoxicam and loxoprofen. The study was a randomized controlled trial that assigned 280 patients to either the TRAM/APAP group or the NSAID group. The TRAM/APAP group had significantly lower pain scores on postoperative days 4, 7, and 14. Also, the TRAM/APAP group achieved independence from ambulatory assistance (cane) significantly faster than the NSAID group. There were no significant differences in motion or length of hospital stay. This study suggests that TRAM/APAP should be considered as a valuable addition to a multimodal pain management regimen. However, tramadol is not without complications and surgeons should be aware of the potential risk for serotonin syndrome associated with tramadol.[34,35] Sternbach[36] reports that serotonin syndrome was originally identified in the 1960s and consists of seratonergic hyperstimulation, which may result in confusion, hypomania, clonus, hypersensitivity, restlessness, shivering, and tremor among other symptoms. Despite the severity of this syndrome, with knowledge of the patient's medication history and the potential drug interactions for medications being used in a multimodal regimen appropriate planning can prevent the development of serotonin syndrome.[37]

Similar to tramadol, tapentadol is also a synthetic opioid that has been shown to be effective and well-tolerated against moderate to severe acute pain and acute postoperative pain.[38] It produces analgesia by acting as a mu-opioid receptor agonist and a norepinephrine reuptake inhibitor.[39] When comparing tapentadol with oxycodone in patients with low back pain or osteoarthritic of the hip/knee, Hale and colleagues[40] reported similar pain relief with less side effects in patients that received tapentadol. Furthermore, when evaluating the use of tapentadol compared with oxycodone in patients with end-stage joint disease of the hip or knee and awaiting joint replacement, Hartrick and colleagues[41] also concluded that tapentadol provided similar pain relief with fewer side effects.

With the emergence of these synthetic analgesics, it seems feasible that one will be able to maintain adequate pain control while decreasing the side effects commonly associated with opioid medications. Thus, the use of these novel medications should be considered in the multimodal pain management model.

ANTICONVULSANTS

Pregabalin (Lyrica) is a structural analogue of γ-aminobutyric acid that acts on voltage gated calcium channels. It was originally introduced in 2004 as an anticonvulsant. Today, it is used to treat epilepsy, neuropathic pain, fibromyalgia, generalized anxiety disorder, and other conditions.[42] Compared with its predecessor, gabapentin, pregabalin has superior oral absorption and bioavailability.[43] Both drugs have received increased interest in recent years as adjuncts in the management of not only neuropathic pain, but also acute postoperative pain.

There have been several studies showing that pregabalin reduces postoperative opioid consumption and reduces postoperative nausea and vomiting. For example, a meta-analysis by Engelman and Cateloy[44] in 2011 evaluated the efficacy and safety of pregabalin for postoperative pain and concluded that the use of pregabalin in the short perioperative time provides additional analgesia, but at the expense of its unique side effects. The study evaluated 18 randomized trials with a total of 1547 patients. The analyzed studies included various surgeries: TKA, lumbar discectomy, thyroidectomy, arthroscopic meniscectomy, among others. The analysis found that pregabalin use decreased the amount of postoperative analgesic drugs. Also, pregabalin resulted in less nausea and vomiting. However, pregabalin increased the risk of dizziness and visual disturbances, known side effects of neuromodulators.

A more recent study on pregabalin by Clarke and colleagues[45] asked whether a perioperative regimen of pregabalin added to the COX-2 inhibitor celecoxib improved pain scores and functional measures 3 months after THA. They randomized 184 patients to receive either pregabalin or placebo, in addition to celecoxib and spinal anesthesia. After surgery, the groups continued to receive either pregabalin or placebo for 7 days after discharge. They found no difference in physical function scores or pain 3 months after surgery. As secondary outcomes, the authors measured acute postoperative pain and adverse effects. The pregabalin group used fewer morphine equivalents (mean, 39.85 mg) than the placebo group (mean, 54.01 mg) in the first 24 hours. Also, pain scores were significantly lower in the pregabalin group for the first week after discharge. The paper concludes that perioperative pregabalin decreased pain and opioid consumption acutely, but does not affect pain or function at 3 months postoperatively.

The effect of pregabalin after TKA has also been recently studied. Dong and colleagues[46] performed a meta-analysis to identify the safety and efficacy of pregabalin versus placebo after TKA and showed significant reductions in pain (at rest and with mobilization) and opioid consumption for the first 48 hours when pregabalin was used as part of a multimodal pain regimen. Moreover, pregabalin decreased the incidence of nausea/vomiting. The study included six trials and 769 patients.

SPINAL ANESTHESIA

Postoperative pain control is affected by the type of anesthesia used for the surgery. Although traditionally general anesthesia was the mainstay for THA and TKA, spinal anesthesia (a form of regional anesthesia) is gaining popularity. Spinal anesthesia provides safe, predictable pain control during and immediately after the operation. Additionally, compared with general anesthesia, spinal anesthesia may lead to less intraoperative blood loss.[47] Finally, when using general anesthesia, the anesthesiologist responds to pain indicators by administering narcotics. In contrast, spinal anesthesia prevents painful stimuli from ever reaching the brain, thereby minimizing pain-induced physiologic responses, such as hypertension and tachycardia. For these reasons, many anesthesiologists and orthopedic surgeons believe that spinal anesthesia should be performed for arthroplasty unless contraindicated.

Contraindications to spinal anesthesia are few, but could include severe degenerative lumbar spine disease or previous spinal fusion surgery. For this reason, surgeons should evaluate the lumbar spine on the preoperative anteroposterior pelvis and long-standing radiographs.

Also, there are some disadvantages associated with spinal anesthesia: possibility of block failure, operating room delays, patient apprehension, and motor blockade preventing same day discharges.

EPIDURAL ANALGESIA

Although it is infrequently used, epidural anesthesia was formerly a popular method of pain control for TKA. A 2003 meta-analysis by Block and coworkers[48] looked at studies on this method of pain control. This review included results from 100 studies, and sought to compare epidural anesthesia with IV opioids. The authors found that regardless of the analgesic agent used or the location of the catheter, epidural anesthesia provided superior postoperative pain control compared with IV opioids.

Epidural anesthesia has significant downsides, however, which have led to its widespread discontinuation Negative aspects of epidural anesthesia include inadvertent motor nerve block, which would delay physical therapy and rehabilitation. Also, numbness in the contralateral lower extremity, ileus, pressure phenomenon, pruritus, epidural hematoma, and nausea/vomiting have been reported. Another drawback of epidural anesthesia is that it limits the options for postoperative prophylaxis against deep venous thrombosis, an important consideration in patients undergoing THA or TKA.

PERIPHERAL NERVE BLOCKS

A peripheral nerve block is a modality of regional anesthesia whereby a local anesthetic is injected around a peripheral nerve, blocking sensory and possibly motor function. Such blocks are becoming increasingly popular for surgeries involving the lower extremity. In general, peripheral nerve blocks are low risk, yet highly effective in managing postoperative pain. Their use is associated with early mobilization, better participation with physical therapy, decreased length of hospital stay, and improved discharge rates from the ambulatory care setting.[49]

An example of a peripheral nerve block used in hip arthroplasty is the fascia iliaca block. This ultrasound-guided block anesthetizes the anterior cutaneous femoral nerve branches and the lateral femoral cutaneous nerve.[50] It is useful for surgery about the proximal femur, including pediatric proximal femur osteotomies, proximal femur fracture fixation, and THA. A recent study by Kearns and coworkers[51] randomized 108

THA patients to receive either a fascia iliaca block or a bolus of spinal morphine with a sham fascia iliaca block. The fascia iliaca group required more IV morphine within the first 24 hours after surgery.

Specific to total knee arthroplasty, Lovald and colleagues[52] showed that early walking reduces the chances of infection, deep venous thrombosis, and arthrofibrosis, the three most common causes of hospital readmission after TKA. Complications associated with peripheral blocks are rare: hematoma formation, systemic toxicity, nerve and vessel damage, and catheter site infection.[53] Additionally, transient muscle weakness and patient falls as a result of this weakness is one of the main concerns associated with peripheral nerve blocks, especially femoral nerve blocks (FNB).[54]

FNB have been one of the most commonly used methods of regional anesthesia for surgery about the knee. The femoral nerve runs under the inguinal ligament, lying lateral to the femoral artery. Its branches innervate the muscles and skin of the anterior compartment of the thigh. In addition to their utility for total knee arthroplasty, FNB was once popular for such surgeries as anterior cruciate ligament reconstruction and fixation of patella fractures.

To examine trends in the use of FNB for knee arthroplasty, Gabriel and colleagues[55] examined the National Anesthesia Clinical Outcomes Registry. From January 2010 to June 2015, there were 219,327 patients in the registry who met inclusion criteria. Of these, 72.7% of patients received an FNB. Younger patients (<18 year old) and patients with higher American Society of Anesthesiologists physical status class (≥III) were less likely to receive an FNB. Also, surgeries performed after 5 PM were less likely to involve an FNB, presumably because the anesthesiologists skilled in regional blockade were no longer available. Cases with an urban zip code had a 20% chance of receiving the block. Despite the high prevalence of FNB cases identified in this registry, contemporary practice is leaning away from the use of FNBs because of concerns associated with quadriceps motor blockade. In the authors' opinion, the best use of femoral nerve catheters may be in the revision setting, when weight-bearing restrictions make the motor blockade moot. Also, in the case of extensor mechanism reconstruction, the patient may benefit from the quadriceps muscle relaxation.

To avoid the quadriceps motor blockade of a FNB, the adductor canal block (ACB) is gaining popularity. The adductor canal lies between the anterior and medial thigh compartments and contains the nerve branch to the vastus medialis and the saphenous nerve, the terminal sensory branch of the femoral nerve. Additionally, an ACB anesthetizes the articular branches of the obturator nerve.[56] This far distally, the femoral nerve has already given off most of its motor branches. As such, blocking the adductor canal can provide similar analgesia to a FNB, while sparing quadriceps function, thereby promoting early ambulation.

In a recent meta-analysis, Jiang and colleagues[57] demonstrated that ACBs resulted in less postoperative opioid consumption than placebo, and less pain at rest and with activities. Most studies comparing ACB and FNB reported similar effects on postoperative pain and opioid consumption. However, the ability to ambulate and quadriceps strength was significantly better in ACB patients. The pooled results indicate that ACB is effective for pain control after TKA.

Both FNBs and ACBs are commonly combined with a posterior block to stop pain stemming from the back of the knee. Formerly, this was done with a separate sciatic nerve block. The disadvantage of blocking the sciatic nerve is its motor blockade, which may cause a foot drop and mask a surgically induced peroneal nerve injury. More recently, the iPACK (infiltration between popliteal artery and capsule of the knee) block has gained popularity, because it only blocks the terminal sensory branches of the tibial nerve. The combination of an ACB and an iPACK is becoming increasingly popular because of its analgesic efficacy and muscle-sparing characteristics. A 2017 paper by Cullom and Weed[58] describes how this combination is especially popular in outpatient TKA surgery.

Fowler and colleagues[59] performed a meta-analysis evaluating epidural analgesia to FNB and concluded that although epidural and FNB provide similar analgesia, the femoral block has a better side effect profile. The analysis included eight randomized trials and 510 patients. Variations on the FNB were used in the reviewed studies: single injection (two studies), femoral catheter (five studies), and lumbar plexus catheter (one study). In addition, three studies included sciatic nerve blockade as an adjunct injection to anesthetize the posterior knee. The results of the study showed no significant difference in pain control, opioid consumption, rehabilitation rates, or nausea/vomiting. The blocked groups did have fewer episodes of hypotension and urinary retention. Also, blocked patients had higher patient satisfaction in two of the three studies that measured this.

One of the prime advantages of peripheral nerve catheters over PCAs and epidural anesthesia is the option for the patient to be discharged with the peripheral catheter still in place and functioning. This strategy can take advantage of the many advantages of earlier hospital discharge, while still ensuring adequate pain control and patient satisfaction. At our institution, Swenson and coworkers[60] has shown that the use of peripheral catheters is associated with few complications (0.3%) in the outpatient setting. In contrast, the risk of oversedation and catheter-site infection associated with PCA and epidural use, respectively, limits their use to the hospital setting only.

Table 1 summarizes the pros and cons of femoral nerve and ACB.

PERIARTICULAR INJECTIONS

In addition to the previously mentioned strategies, PAIs is another tool in the multimodal analgesia armamentarium. PAIs are performed by the surgeon, usually near the conclusion of the arthroplasty procedure. Compared with the femoral and ACB, PAIs work earlier in the pain pathway, at the site of primary tissue damage. Usually, a combination of the following substances has been used in a PAI cocktail: opioids, NSAIDs, local anesthetics, antibiotics, clonidine, and epinephrine. The cocktail is injected into tissues that are believed to cause significant pain postoperatively. In TKA, for example, Guild and coworkers[61] discuss the neuroanatomy about the knee and describe an injection technique for treating the periarticular regions with increased neurosensory perception.

In a 2015 study, Vaishya and colleagues[62] randomized 80 TKA patients to receive a PAI of either a cocktail of medicines (morphine, ketorolac, bupivacaine, and adrenaline) or normal saline and report less PCA narcotics and lower pain during rest and activity in the treatment group. Moreover, this group had greater patient satisfaction scores. There were no complications related to the injections.

To compare PAI with FNB, Kurosaka and colleagues[63] randomized 45 TKA patients to receive either PAI or FNB. Their PAI cocktail consisted of ketoprofen, ropivacaine, epinephrine, and normal saline. The FNB consisted of a ropivacaine loading dose, with continuous infusion for 48 hours after. The PAI group had lower pain scores at rest on postoperative Day 1, but pain scores were similar thereafter. The PAI group also consumed fewer opioids in the initial 24 hours. There were no differences in functional recovery or complications. The authors advocated for the use of PAI over FNB for TKA.

More recently, to prolong the effect of the PAI, LB has been used as a component of PAI cocktails. LB is a novel bupivacaine formulation that has been reported to last up to 72 hours.[64] Several studies have established the safety and efficacy of LB.[65,66] For example, a 2017 paper by McGraw-Tatum and coworkers[67] found that fascia iliaca blocks and LB provide excellent pain control after THA. Despite this, there are a myriad of studies demonstrating conflicting outcomes and further research is needed to determine if the proposed benefits justify the cost of LB.

AUTHORS' RECOMMENDATIONS AND STRATEGIES

The data supporting multimodal pain management for THA and TKA are compelling. As such, the authors work closely with our anesthesiology colleagues to fine tune multimodal protocols for preoperative, intraoperative, and postoperative analgesia. Our current protocol is found in Fig. 1. The implementation of a multimodal approach, in addition to earlier initiation of physical therapy, has allowed us to improve

| Table 1 | | |
| Femoral nerve and adductor canal blocks for total knee arthroplasty | | |
Peripheral Block	Pros	Cons
Femoral nerve	Easier to perform Better proximal thigh analgesia	Quadriceps motor blockade • Delays walking • Increases fall risk • Requires the use of a knee immobilizer
Adductor canal	No quadriceps motor blockade	More difficult to perform Less proximal thigh analgesia

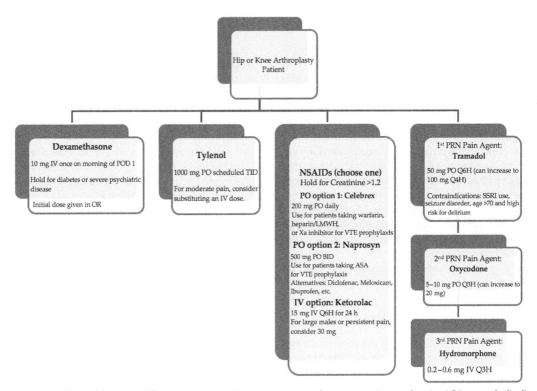

Fig. 1. A multimodal protocol for preoperative, intraoperative, and postoperative analgesia. ASA, acetylsalicylic acid; LMWH, low-molecular-weight heparin; OR, operating room; SSRI, selective serotonin reuptake inhibitor; VTE, venous thromboembolism.

pain scores, opioid consumption, walking distance, and length of stay.[68,69]

SUMMARY

THA and TKA are associated with significant perioperative pain. Furthermore, uncontrolled pain can adversely affect recovery by increasing the risk of complications, the length of stay, and cost. Pain also detracts from patient satisfaction, which results in decreased hospital and physician reimbursements. Historically, opioids were the mainstay of perioperative pain control. However, opioids are associated with significant downsides including respiratory depression, constipation, and dependence. As such, the pre-emptive use of a multimodal pain management approach has become the standard of care to manage pain after hip and knee arthroplasty. Multimodal pain management uses oral medicines (eg, COX-2 inhibitors, neuromodulators), peripheral nerve blocks, intra-articular injections, and other tools to reduce the need for opioids. The use a multimodal approach promises to decrease complications, improve outcomes, and increase patient satisfaction after hip and knee arthroplasty.

REFERENCES

1. Lawrence RC, Felson DT, Helmick CG, et al. Estimates of the prevalence of arthritis and other rheumatic conditions in the United States. Part II. Arthritis Rheum 2008;58(1):26–35.
2. Trousdale RT, McGrory BJ, Berry DJ, et al. Patients' concerns prior to undergoing total hip and total knee arthroplasty. Mayo Clin Proc 1999;74(10): 978–82.
3. Parvizi J. Pain management following total joint arthroplasty: making strides. J Bone Joint Surg Am 2012;94(16):1441.
4. Merskey H. Logic, truth and language in concepts of pain. Qual Life Res 1994;3(Suppl 1):S69–76.
5. Dalury DF, Lieberman JR, Macdonald SJ. Current and innovative pain management techniques in total knee arthroplasty. Instr Course Lect 2012;61: 383–8.
6. Riddle DL, Wade JB, Jiranek WA, et al. Preoperative pain catastrophizing predicts pain outcome after knee arthroplasty. Clin Orthop Relat Res 2010; 468(3):798–806.
7. Sinatra RS, Torres J, Bustos AM. Pain management after major orthopaedic surgery: current strategies and new concepts. J Am Acad Orthop Surg 2002; 10(2):117–29.

8. Macintyre PE. Safety and efficacy of patient-controlled analgesia. Br J Anaesth 2001;87(1):36–46.

9. Kastanias P, Gowans S, Tumber PS, et al. Patient-controlled oral analgesia for postoperative pain management following total knee replacement. Pain Res Manag 2010;15(1):11–6.

10. Dominick KL, Bosworth HB, Dudley TK, et al. Patterns of opioid analgesic prescription among patients with osteoarthritis. J pain Palliat Care Pharmacother 2004;18(1):31–46.

11. Halawi MJ, Vovos TJ, Green CL, et al. Opioid-based analgesia: impact on total joint arthroplasty. J Arthroplasty 2015;30(12):2360–3.

12. Wheeler M, Oderda GM, Ashburn MA, et al. Adverse events associated with postoperative opioid analgesia: a systematic review. J Pain 2002;3(3):159–80.

13. Scuderi GR. The challenges of perioperative pain management in total joint arthroplasty. Am J Orthop (Belle Mead NJ) 2015;44(10 Suppl):S2–4.

14. Sing DC, Barry JJ, Cheah JW, et al. Long-acting opioid use independently predicts perioperative complication in total joint arthroplasty. J Arthroplasty 2016;31(9 Suppl):170–4.e1.

15. Nguyen LC, Sing DC, Bozic KJ. Preoperative reduction of opioid use before total joint arthroplasty. J Arthroplasty 2016;31(9 Suppl):282–7.

16. Wall PD. The prevention of postoperative pain. Pain 1988;33(3):289–90.

17. Kehlet H, Dahl JB. The value of "multimodal" or "balanced analgesia" in postoperative pain treatment. Anesth Analg 1993;77(5):1048–56.

18. Dahl JB, Kehlet H. The value of pre-emptive analgesia in the treatment of postoperative pain. Br J Anaesth 1993;70(4):434–9.

19. Diaz-Heredia J, Loza E, Cebreiro I, et al. Preventive analgesia in hip or knee arthroplasty: a systematic review. Rev Esp Cir Ortop Traumatol 2015;59(2):73–90.

20. Remerand F, Le Tendre C, Baud A, et al. The early and delayed analgesic effects of ketamine after total hip arthroplasty: a prospective, randomized, controlled, double-blind study. Anesth Analg 2009;109(6):1963–71.

21. Min BW, Kim Y, Cho HM, et al. Perioperative pain management in total hip arthroplasty: Korean Hip Society guidelines. Hip Pelvis 2016;28(1):15–23.

22. Gibbons CE, Solan MC, Ricketts DM, et al. Cryotherapy compared with Robert Jones bandage after total knee replacement: a prospective randomized trial. Int Orthop 2001;25(4):250–2.

23. Healy WL, Seidman J, Pfeifer BA, et al. Cold compressive dressing after total knee arthroplasty. Clin Orthop Relat Res 1994;(299):143–6.

24. Toms L, McQuay HJ, Derry S, et al. Single dose oral paracetamol (acetaminophen) for postoperative pain in adults. Cochrane Database Syst Rev 2008;(4):CD004602.

25. Politi JR, Davis RL 2nd, Matrka AK. Randomized prospective trial comparing the use of intravenous versus oral acetaminophen in total joint arthroplasty. J Arthroplasty 2016;32(4):1125–7.

26. Kelly JS, Opsha Y, Costello J, et al. Opioid use in knee arthroplasty after receiving intravenous acetaminophen. Pharmacotherapy 2014;34(Suppl 1):22S–6S.

27. Jibril F, Sharaby S, Mohamed A, et al. Intravenous versus oral acetaminophen for pain: systematic review of current evidence to support clinical decision-making. Can J Hosp Pharm 2015;68(3):238–47.

28. Buvanendran A, Kroin JS, Berger RA, et al. Upregulation of prostaglandin E2 and interleukins in the central nervous system and peripheral tissue during and after surgery in humans. Anesthesiology 2006;104(3):403–10.

29. Robinson CM, Christie J, Malcolm-Smith N. Nonsteroidal antiinflammatory drugs, perioperative blood loss, and transfusion requirements in elective hip arthroplasty. J Arthroplasty 1993;8(6):607–10.

30. Teerawattananon C, Tantayakom P, Suwanawiboon B, et al. Risk of perioperative bleeding related to highly selective cyclooxygenase-2 inhibitors: a systematic review and meta-analysis. Semin Arthritis Rheum 2017;46(4):520–8.

31. Buvanendran A, Kroin JS, Tuman KJ, et al. Effects of perioperative administration of a selective cyclooxygenase 2 inhibitor on pain management and recovery of function after knee replacement: a randomized controlled trial. JAMA 2003;290(18):2411–8.

32. Dayer P, Collart L, Desmeules J. The pharmacology of tramadol. Drugs 1994;47(Suppl 1):3–7.

33. Mochizuki T, Yano K, Ikari K, et al. Tramadol hydrochloride/acetaminophen combination versus nonsteroidal anti-inflammatory drug for the treatment of perioperative pain after total knee arthroplasty: a prospective, randomized, open-label clinical trial. J Orthop Sci 2016;21(5):625–9.

34. Kitson R, Carr B. Tramadol and severe serotonin syndrome. Anaesthesia 2005;60(9):934–5.

35. Spiller HA, Gorman SE, Villalobos D, et al. Prospective multicenter evaluation of tramadol exposure. J Toxicol Clin Toxicol 1997;35(4):361–4.

36. Sternbach H. The serotonin syndrome. Am J Psychiatry 1991;148(6):705–13.

37. Dvir Y, Smallwood P. Serotonin syndrome: a complex but easily avoidable condition. Gen Hosp Psychiatry 2008;30(3):284–7.

38. Pierce DM, Shipstone E. Pharmacology update: tapentadol for neuropathic pain. Am J Hosp Palliat Care 2012;29(8):663–6.

39. Wade WE, Spruill WJ. Tapentadol hydrochloride: a centrally acting oral analgesic. Clin Ther 2009; 31(12):2804–18.

40. Hale M, Upmalis D, Okamoto A, et al. Tolerability of tapentadol immediate release in patients with lower back pain or osteoarthritis of the hip or knee over 90 days: a randomized, double-blind study. Curr Med Res Opin 2009;25(5):1095–104.

41. Hartrick C, Van Hove I, Stegmann JU, et al. Efficacy and tolerability of tapentadol immediate release and oxycodone HCl immediate release in patients awaiting primary joint replacement surgery for end-stage joint disease: a 10-day, phase III, randomized, double-blind, active- and placebo-controlled study. Clin Ther 2009;31(2):260–71.

42. Dworkin RH, Kirkpatrick P. Pregabalin. Nat Rev Drug Discov 2005;4(6):455–6.

43. Bockbrader HN, Wesche D, Miller R, et al. A comparison of the pharmacokinetics and pharmacodynamics of pregabalin and gabapentin. Clin Pharmacokinet 2010;49(10):661–9.

44. Engelman E, Cateloy F. Efficacy and safety of perioperative pregabalin for post-operative pain: a meta-analysis of randomized-controlled trials. Acta Anaesthesiol Scand 2011;55(8):927–43.

45. Clarke H, Page GM, McCartney CJ, et al. Pregabalin reduces postoperative opioid consumption and pain for 1 week after hospital discharge, but does not affect function at 6 weeks or 3 months after total hip arthroplasty. Br J Anaesth 2015;115(6):903–11.

46. Dong J, Li W, Wang Y. The effect of pregabalin on acute postoperative pain in patients undergoing total knee arthroplasty: a meta-analysis. Int J Surg 2016;34:148–60.

47. Rashiq S, Finegan BA. The effect of spinal anesthesia on blood transfusion rate in total joint arthroplasty. Can J Surg 2006;49(6):391–6.

48. Block BM, Liu SS, Rowlingson AJ, et al. Efficacy of postoperative epidural analgesia: a meta-analysis. JAMA 2003;290(18):2455–63.

49. Stein BE, Srikumaran U, Tan EW, et al. Lower-extremity peripheral nerve blocks in the perioperative pain management of orthopaedic patients: AAOS exhibit selection. J Bone Joint Surg Am 2012; 94(22):e167.

50. Bullock WM, Yalamuri SM, Gregory SH, et al. Ultrasound-guided suprainguinal fascia iliaca technique provides benefit as an analgesic adjunct for patients undergoing total hip arthroplasty. J Ultrasound Med 2017;36(2):433–8.

51. Kearns R, Macfarlane A, Grant A, et al. A randomised, controlled, double blind, non-inferiority trial of ultrasound-guided fascia iliaca block vs. spinal morphine for analgesia after primary hip arthroplasty. Anaesthesia 2016;71(12):1431–40.

52. Lovald ST, Ong KL, Lau EC, et al. Readmission and complications for catheter and injection femoral nerve block administration after total knee arthroplasty in the Medicare population. J Arthroplasty 2015;30(12):2076–81.

53. Howell R, Hill B, Hoffman C, et al. Peripheral nerve blocks for surgery about the knee. JBJS Rev 2016; 4(12) [pii:01874474-201612000-00003].

54. Pelt CE, Anderson AW, Anderson MB, et al. Postoperative falls after total knee arthroplasty in patients with a femoral nerve catheter: can we reduce the incidence? J Arthroplasty 2014;29(6):1154–7.

55. Gabriel RA, Kaye AD, Nagrebetsky A, et al. Utilization of femoral nerve blocks for total knee arthroplasty. J Arthroplasty 2016;31(8):1680–5.

56. Kapoor R, Adhikary SD, Siefring C, et al. The saphenous nerve and its relationship to the nerve to the vastus medialis in and around the adductor canal: an anatomical study. Acta Anaesthesiol Scand 2012;56(3):365–7.

57. Jiang X, Wang QQ, Wu CA, et al. Analgesic efficacy of adductor canal block in total knee arthroplasty: a meta-analysis and systematic review. Orthop Surg 2016;8(3):294–300.

58. Cullom C, Weed JT. Anesthetic and analgesic management for outpatient knee arthroplasty. Curr Pain Headache Rep 2017;21(5):23.

59. Fowler SJ, Symons J, Sabato S, et al. Epidural analgesia compared with peripheral nerve blockade after major knee surgery: a systematic review and meta-analysis of randomized trials. Br J Anaesth 2008;100(2):154–64.

60. Swenson JD, Bay N, Loose E, et al. Outpatient management of continuous peripheral nerve catheters placed using ultrasound guidance: an experience in 620 patients. Anesth Analg 2006;103(6):1436–43.

61. Guild GN 3rd, Galindo RP, Marino J, et al. Periarticular regional analgesia in total knee arthroplasty: a review of the neuroanatomy and injection technique. Orthop Clin North Am 2015;46(1):1–8.

62. Vaishya R, Wani AM, Vijay V. Local infiltration analgesia reduces pain and hospital stay after primary TKA: randomized controlled double blind trial. Acta Orthop Belg 2015;81(4):720–9.

63. Kurosaka K, Tsukada S, Seino D, et al. Local infiltration analgesia versus continuous femoral nerve block in pain relief after total knee arthroplasty: a randomized controlled trial. J Arthroplasty 2016; 31(4):913–7.

64. Bramlett K, Onel E, Viscusi ER, et al. A randomized, double-blind, dose-ranging study comparing wound infiltration of DepoFoam bupivacaine, an extended-release liposomal bupivacaine, to bupivacaine HCl for postsurgical analgesia in total knee arthroplasty. Knee 2012;19(5):530–6.

65. Tong YC, Kaye AD, Urman RD. Liposomal bupivacaine and clinical outcomes. Best Pract Res Clin Anaesthesiol 2014;28(1):15–27.

66. Viscusi ER, Sinatra R, Onel E, et al. The safety of liposome bupivacaine, a novel local analgesic formulation. Clin J pain 2014;30(2):102–10.

67. McGraw-Tatum MA, Groover MT, George NE, et al. A prospective, randomized trial comparing liposomal bupivacaine vs fascia iliaca compartment block for postoperative pain control in total hip arthroplasty. J Arthroplasty 2017;32:2181–5.

68. Pelt CE, Anderson MB, Pendleton R, et al. Improving value in primary total joint arthroplasty care pathways: changes in inpatient physical therapy staffing. Arthroplasty Today 2017;3(1):45–9.

69. Peters CL, Shirley B, Erickson J. The effect of a new multimodal perioperative anesthetic regimen on postoperative pain, side effects, rehabilitation, and length of hospital stay after total joint arthroplasty. J Arthroplasty 2006;21(6 Suppl 2):132–8.

Patient Satisfaction After Total Knee Arthroplasty
A Realistic or Imaginary Goal?

Emmanuel Gibon, MD, PhD, Marla J. Goodman, BA, MA (Int Rel),
Stuart B. Goodman, MD, PhD*

KEYWORDS

• Patient satisfaction • Knee arthroplasty • Patient expectations • Outcomes

KEY POINTS

- There is no consensus on the optimal method of ensuring or measuring patient satisfaction. Many studies show that there is no association between patients' experiences and the quality of health care.
- The general states of preoperative physical and mental health are highly correlated with patient satisfaction and outcome after surgery. Patients with preoperative health issues such as mild to moderate arthritis have a higher risk of dissatisfaction after total knee arthroplasty (TKA) surgery.
- The surgical approach plays a minor role for long-term satisfaction after TKA.
- Perioperative pain control, postoperative rehabilitation, and outcome/satisfaction after TKA are clearly linked. Patients with uncontrolled pain do not participate fully in their postoperative exercises, do not obtain maximal function, and therefore become dissatisfied with their operations.

PATIENT SATISFACTION AFTER TOTAL KNEE ARTHROPLASTY

This article is designed to help physicians understand that:

- Patient expectations are often varied, and in some cases there is no correlation between fulfillment of patient expectations and patient satisfaction.
- A variety of different factors determine the degree of patient satisfaction after total knee arthroplasty (TKA).
- Patients with other musculoskeletal issues, such as low back pain or pain in other joints, also have a higher risk of being disappointed.

- A TKA performed in patients with isolated and less destabilizing knee osteoarthritis carries the risk of dissatisfaction.
- Patient satisfaction after TKA seems to be strongly correlated with the fulfillment of the preoperative expectations.
- The amount of flexion needed to accomplish most activities of daily living is controversial.
- High-flexion devices may result in less polyethylene stress and lower patellar ligament strains, which may result in better function and long-term survivorship; however, the effects on patient satisfaction are unknown.

Funding Sources: No funding sources for this article.
Conflict of Interest: The authors declare no conflict of interest.
Department of Orthopaedic Surgery, Stanford University, 300 Pasteur Drive, Edwards Building R116, Stanford, CA 94305, USA
* Corresponding author. Department of Orthopaedic Surgery, 450 Broadway Street, M/C 6342, Redwood City, CA 94063.
E-mail address: goodbone@stanford.edu

Orthop Clin N Am 48 (2017) 421–431
http://dx.doi.org/10.1016/j.ocl.2017.06.001
0030-5898/17/© 2017 Elsevier Inc. All rights reserved.

- Patients are more satisfied when their pain is controlled adequately after surgery.
- Perioperative pain control, postoperative rehabilitation, and outcome/satisfaction after TKA are clearly linked.

INTRODUCTION

A recent trend in American health care delivery is the emphasis on patient satisfaction. However, patient expectations are often varied, and in some cases there is no correlation between fulfillment of patient expectations and patient satisfaction.[1] Although the outcome of treatment and degree of recovery of patients are of the utmost importance, there is no consensus on the optimal method of ensuring or measuring patient satisfaction. Many studies show that there is no association between patients' experiences and the quality of health care[2]; in some cases, an overemphasis on patient satisfaction can come at the expense of patient health care. In one study, patient satisfaction and health were not clearly correlated; the most satisfied patients had a 26% higher mortality risk.[3] Some hospitals and health care providers seem to put too much emphasis on making health care sound better in order to get higher ratings.[4]

One example in which clinical outcome and patient satisfaction can be disparate is TKA. TKA is currently one of the most safe, efficacious, and cost-effective operations in all of surgery, and is performed worldwide.[5,6] However, up to 20% of patients report long-term pain after TKA, which is dramatically more than after total hip arthroplasty (THA).[7,8] As shown by Nashi and colleagues,[9] 31.1% and 28.9% of patients experience residual knee pain at 1 and 2 years respectively after TKA. Moreover, there is poorer restoration of functional outcome after TKA compared with THA.[10] Despite these observations, the critical factors influencing patient satisfaction after TKA remain controversial. A variety of different factors determine the degree of patient satisfaction after TKA, and many of these factors are contradictory or not within the surgeon's scope of care or control. This article examines some of the primary considerations and determinants associated with patient satisfaction after TKA. The factors that seem to affect patient satisfaction can be grouped into different categories, including:

1. Patient-associated factors
2. Surgical factors
3. Prosthesis characteristics
4. Perioperative factors
5. Factors associated with nursing and general medical care

METHODS

The authors performed a Medline search using the following key words: total knee arthroplasty or total knee replacement, outcome, and satisfaction. All relevant articles published over the last 15 years were considered for inclusion. Abstracts and, where relevant, complete articles were examined and assessed for patient inclusion criteria, outcome variables, and measures of satisfaction used. Review articles were read and references examined for additional articles to include. Fully published articles of clinical series with data were included in this review, and the investigators' observations and conclusions summarized. Several relevant opinion editorials were also reviewed to guide the discussion.

RESULTS

After review and analysis, the present authors realized that the primary factors that affect patient satisfaction could be grouped into 5 different categories:

1. Patient-associated factors
2. Surgical factors
3. Prosthesis characteristics
4. Perioperative factors
5. Factors associated with nursing and general medical care

Table 1 summarizes the conclusions for each of the factors.

Patient-associated Factors
Issues related to the patients' preoperative and postoperative physical and mental states
The general states of preoperative physical and mental health are highly correlated with patient satisfaction and outcome after surgery. Patients with preoperative health issues such as mild to moderate arthritis have a higher risk of dissatisfaction after TKA surgery.[11] This finding does not represent an indictment but surgeons should inform those patients about the increased dissatisfaction risk. Patients who have disproportional pain to the radiographic findings may not have the same outcomes and satisfaction, mainly because of higher sensitivity to pain. Patients with other musculoskeletal issues, such as low back pain or pain in other joints, also have a higher risk of being disappointed. These

Table 1
Factors affecting patient satisfaction after total knee arthroplasty

Primary Factors	Details	Effect on Satisfaction
Patient-associated factors	Associated musculoskeletal issues	↑ Dissatisfaction
	Self-reported allergies	↑ Dissatisfaction
	Isolated and less destabilizing knee osteoarthritis	↑ Dissatisfaction
	Knee-related issues for a longer period	↑ Satisfaction
	Fulfillment of preoperative expectations	↑ Satisfaction
	Educational classes	↑ Satisfaction
	Patient age	Controversial
Surgical factors	Surgical approach	Controversial
	Alignment	Controversial
Prosthesis factors	High-flexion implants	Controversial
	Flexion needed to accomplish most activities	Controversial
Perioperative factors	Efficient pain management	↑ Satisfaction
	Poststructured postoperative exercise programs	↑ Satisfaction
Factors associated with nursing and general medical care	Higher level of general care	↑ Satisfaction
	Decreased length of hospital stay	↑ Satisfaction

patients showed less improvement after undergoing TKA with regard to perceived physical well-being. Other factors for high risk of dissatisfaction include increasing age and heart disease[12] as well as sensitivity to pain, fibromyalgia, and patient-related factors that lead to complications and dissatisfaction, such as smoking, drug abuse, obesity, and diabetes. Patients with low back pain were more likely to be dissatisfied with their TKA, irrespective of their preoperative mental well-being. In one study, patients with no back pain had a postoperative score of 41.8 on the Medical Outcomes Study Short Form 12 (SF-12) Physical Health Composite Scale (PCS) and a score of 52.4 on the SF-12 Mental Health Composite Scale (MCS). In contrast, patients with back pain had scores of 35.5 and 48.5 on the SF-12 PCS and MCS respectively.[13] Patients with self-reported allergies reported lower levels of satisfaction after undergoing TKA, as shown by McLawhorn and colleagues.[14] The investigators state that patient-reported allergies are a criterion for somatoform disorders, which may explain the lower levels of satisfaction associated with those allergies.

If a patient's general health degraded after their TKA, the patient was less likely to be satisfied with the knee procedure. In one study, out of 2350 patients who underwent primary unilateral TKA, 7.2% of patients reported no change and 2.3% of patients reported a worsening of

their quality of life at 2 years postoperatively. Higher baseline levels of quality-of-life scores for pain, stiffness, and function were associated with less reported improvement after surgery, which means that a TKA performed in patients with isolated and less destabilizing knee osteoarthritis carries the risk of dissatisfaction. This finding shows how unrelated health issues can have a negative impact on patient satisfaction after a specific operation.[15] In contrast, patients who have knee-related issues for a longer period of time, such as chronic disease, are more likely to be satisfied after undergoing knee surgery. For example, in one study in Sweden, only 14% of 3203 patients with rheumatoid arthritis were dissatisfied, whereas 30% of 191 patients with osteonecrosis were dissatisfied.[16]

Expectations
Patient satisfaction after TKA seems to be strongly correlated with the fulfillment of the preoperative expectations. In one study, a group 4709 patients received hip and knee replacements; before the surgery they completed patient-reported outcome measurement questionnaires, Oxford Hip or Knee Scores, and SF-12s health assessments as well as follow-up questionnaires after 6 and 12 months. Final patient satisfaction and meeting expectations had an r value of .74, with a statistical significance of less than 0.001 (which means there is a high correlation).[17] The r value, also referred to as

the Pearson r, is a measure of linear correlation. The value ranges from −1 (negative linear correlation) to +1 (positive linear correlation). In contrast, a literature review that analyzed the results of 5 studies on patient satisfaction after TKA found that there was no significant relationship between expectations and satisfaction in the 2 studies that included this facet of satisfaction.[18] Patients who had unrealistic expectations, like those who thought they could engage in strenuous activity 12 months after their surgery, were less satisfied. In this particular study, strenuous activity was calculated by multiplying the average hours of activity per week by the activity's metabolic equivalent, and baseline activity was measured using the Historical Leisure Activity questionnaire.[19]

Another key issue related to expectations is pain anticipated after surgery. In one study, patients who had levels of pain that were within their levels of expectation were satisfied overall. The patients were asked what their expectations were with regard to pain, and these were graded on a 4-point Likert scale. After 6 months, the patients were asked whether their expectations had been fulfilled with regard to pain, limitations of activities, and overall success of the surgery.[20] In another study, 1 group of patients was debriefed verbally and given an information leaflet describing what they could expect from the surgery with regard to pain, pain management, physiotherapy, and the importance of taking an active role in communicating their symptoms with staff. The patients in the treatment group all stated that they were satisfied or very satisfied with their pain management, whereas the patients in the control group were more dissatisfied.[21] Such a result emphasizes the importance of preoperative joint conferences and educational classes.

Patient age

In some studies, increased age was positively correlated with higher patient satisfaction whereas in other studies, the opposite was true. For example, in 1 study, older patients were less satisfied with their surgeries overall, possibly caused by/because of higher complication rates.[22] In contrast, another study found that older patients were more satisfied with their TKAs. Patients 55 years old and younger, patients between the ages of 55 and 64 years, and patients more than the age of 65 years had mean satisfaction scores of 7.1, 7.7, and 8.3 respectively. Notably, satisfaction clearly increased with age, most likely because younger patients had higher expectations with regard to

their recovery time and subsequent activity level.[23] Similarly, in one study featuring 45 men and 35 women aged 41 to 89 years, younger men had higher (and perhaps unrealistic) expectations regarding the outcome of their surgery and were less satisfied than women. In this study, 71 implants were cemented posterior cruciate-retaining prostheses, 6 were cemented posterior-stabilized prosthesis, and the remaining 3 were a Press-Fit condylar system.[24] In other studies, age had no effect on patient satisfaction. For instance, one study outlined how, in a study of 989 TKAs in 755 patients (248 male, 507 female), satisfied patients were 65.1 ± 8.9 years old, and dissatisfied patients were 64.3 ± 10 years old.[25] Thus, there is no uniformly conclusive evidence showing that age is a factor in one way or another.

Surgical Factors

Surgical factors such as anatomic approach for TKA, minimally invasive surgery, and overall limb alignment have a bearing on patients' satisfaction with their surgical procedures.

Surgical approach

Although different so-called minimally invasive surgical approaches are currently used for TKA, there is limited high-quality scientific evidence supporting improved outcome or patient satisfaction with their use. In a recent review, Costa and colleagues[26] examined all level I and II data on surgical approach and outcome for TKA. The minimidvastus surgical approach seemed to have improved quadriceps muscle function at 1 and 3 months, and fewer complications compared with other minimally invasive and standard approaches. The minimally invasive lateral approach had the highest complication rate. In another systemic review and meta-analysis, the subvastus but not minimidvastus approach had a shorter hospital stay and decreased blood loss compared with the medial parapatellar approach. The medial parapatellar approach was also associated with a longer period to straight-leg raising. Range of motion was similar with all 3 approaches at 1 year.[27] A prospective randomized study comparing the subvastus and midvastus approaches showed no differences in operative time, total blood loss, straight-leg-raising test, range of motion, or patient preference at 3 months and 2 years.[28] In a prospective study of bilateral TKA comparing the medial parapatellar approach in one knee and the minimidvastus approach in the other, in a comprehensive analysis involving pain score determination, patient preference, gait analysis, and strength testing, the only significant difference was increased isokinetic and isometric extension torque at 3 weeks in the minimidvastus group.[29] In addition, a meta-analysis of 18 randomized clinical trials comparing the minimidvastus surgical approach with the standard medial parapatellar approach showed improvements in pain and range of motion at 1 to 2 weeks with the former, but no other differences in the myriad of other outcome variables measured between 6 weeks and 1 year. However, the minimidvastus approach took longer to perform.[30] Therefore, the surgical approach plays a minor role for long-term satisfaction after TKA.

Alignment

Most surgeons soon realize that patients are displeased with residual deformity after total knee replacement has been performed. Despite this logical observation, few studies have reported data to substantiate it. In a retrospective review of 500 TKAs in Japanese patients with a minimum follow-up of 2 years, Matsuda and colleagues[22] found that residual postoperative varus alignment and advanced age negatively affected patient satisfaction. In another study, 23% of Canadian patients were dissatisfied with their limb alignments after TKA, and had a poorer perception of their pain and range of motion, even though their Knee Society and Oxford Knee Scores were similar to those who were satisfied with their alignment.[31] The current clinical scores therefore have a ceiling effect and cannot accurately capture patient-relevant outcomes.

Prosthesis Characteristics
How much knee flexion is needed in daily life?

The amount of flexion needed to accomplish most activities of daily living is controversial. One study noted that patients only flexed their knees more than 90° 0.5% of the time.[32] However, 135° of flexion seems to be needed for all daily activities in Western cultures.[33] Perhaps even less flexion, 128° to 132°, is sufficient.[34] In another study, range of motion was only ranked as the ninth most important factor related to patient satisfaction after TKA; other activities (such as climbing stairs) were considered to be of greater importance.[35] In India, where squatting and other high-flexion activities are more common, one study concluded (surprisingly) that "deep knee flexion is not an essential prerequisite for patient satisfaction after total knee replacement."[20] Furthermore, daily activity

(with regard to exercise) had no impact on patient satisfaction.[36]

High-flexion implants

Most conventional TKAs result in flexion of approximately 100° to 115°, which is sufficient to accomplish virtually all activities of daily living (83° of flexion is needed to climb stairs, 90° to descend stairs, and 93° to rise from a chair). However, now that TKAs are being performed in younger, more active individuals, there is a desire to obtain even more flexion by some. This extra flexion may be even more important in societies in which squatting and specific methods of kneeling and sitting are everyday occurrences. High flexion (the ability to bend the knee >130°) is a recent trend both in terms of new knee replacements and general postoperative function. Several studies have shown that a single-design, high-flexion, mobile-bearing, posterior-stabilized knee resulted in less pain and higher overall satisfaction. In one study, the flexion obtained varied from 85° to 155°.[37] However, in another study, patients who received a standard prosthesis and those who received a high-flexion prosthesis had similar satisfaction with regard to pain and clinical outcome of surgery.[38] Higher flexion did not have any correlation with overall patient satisfaction in several other studies.[39] Moreover, no differences were found in average knee flexion between patients with high-flexion and standard TKAs.[40] High-flexion devices may result in less polyethylene stress and lower patellar ligament strains, which may result in better function and long-term survivorship; however, the effects on patient satisfaction are unknown.[41] Nashi and colleagues[9] showed that patients with posterior-stabilized implants had better functional outcomes at 2 years.

Perioperative Factors
Pain protocols

Various different protocols have been described to mitigate pain during and even after discharge after TKA. Spinal or general anesthesia is often supplemented with peripheral nerve blocks, including femoral nerve or adductor canal block, and sciatic nerve block. Various different pain cocktails have been injected or infused (such as steroidal and nonsteroidal medication, narcotics, and local anesthetics), and often these are supplemented with oral medication (such as cyclooxygenase-2 inhibitors, acetaminophen, and membrane stabilizing drugs).[42–48] The aim is to minimize the adverse effects from the consumption of systemic and oral narcotics. There have been few prospective randomized studies to identify which pain cocktail is best; however, patients are distinctly more satisfied when their pain is controlled adequately after surgery.[49–51]

Postoperative rehabilitation

Perioperative pain control, postoperative rehabilitation, and outcome/satisfaction after TKA are clearly linked. Patients with uncontrolled pain do not participate fully in their postoperative exercises, do not obtain maximal function, and therefore become dissatisfied with their operations. A structured postoperative exercise program seems to facilitate functional recovery.[52–54] There is little evidence to support the use of continuous passive motion perioperatively; however, patients frequently request its use,[55] although its effect remains controversial.[56,57]

Factors Associated with Nursing and General Medical Care

Hospital care

Patients who rate their hospital care highly have higher scores on their health-related quality of life up to 1 year after their surgery. This finding shows that immediate postoperative satisfaction (related to all aspects of patient care, not just the surgery) influences patient satisfaction.[58] One good example of this is how changes in policy in Ontario, Canada, negatively influenced patient satisfaction after their second joint replacements. Changes reduced wait times, lengths of hospital stay, and physio-therapy access. Even though wait times for surgery were decreased overall, perceived wait time was still high, because patients calculated their wait times from the onset of illness until final treatment, as opposed to starting after the first surgical consultation.[59] Some studies[60–64] compared clinical outcomes for TKA performed in outpatient settings versus inpatient settings. Among them, only the work of Kolisek and colleagues[64] assessed the satisfaction criterion. The investigators found no difference for satisfaction between outpatient and inpatient settings for TKA.

Postoperative care/length of hospital stay

Postoperative care during rehabilitation is also a key factor in patient satisfaction. In one study, patient satisfaction increased when continuous passive motion units were ready for patient use. In the same study, rehabilitation staff received specialized training in how to care for patients with joint replacements, which also led to a higher level of care.[65] Patients were discharged 1 day earlier, and received 1 day less

of postoperative care. In another study, patients who remained in the hospital longer after surgery were less satisfied, although it is difficult to pinpoint the exact cause of this dissatisfaction.[15] Furthermore, postoperative performance is not always correlated with patient satisfaction. Often, happy patients and unhappy patients had similar clinical findings, performance tests, and radiographic results. Even if there was no need for revision surgery, unhappy patients continued to show more pain on the visual analog scale and hospital anxiety and depression scale.[66]

Even different postoperative forms have varying effects on patients' reported self-satisfaction. Patients reported higher levels of satisfaction when a change in the reporting mechanism was instituted, and this did not in reality reflect any significant change.[67] Furthermore, when patients were asked open-ended questions regarding their satisfaction, the responses tended to be more negative compared with closed questions.[68]

DISCUSSION

The number of TKAs performed in the United States is rapidly increasing. By the year 2020, the number of primary TKAs is projected to exceed 1.5 million cases per year.[69] TKA is a safe and efficacious operation that relieves pain and improves function. Originally, this operation was intended for elderly patients with severe end-stage rheumatoid or osteoarthritis. However, more recently, TKA has been extended to younger, more active patients with higher demands in lifestyle. This change has presented challenges for all parties concerned with the delivery of health care, including patients, doctors and allied health care workers, hospitals, and payers. After reconstructive operations such as TKA, patients have high expectations of resuming a normal lifestyle with little down time, expense, pain, and suffering. Health care workers, hospitals, and payers aspire to deliver high-quality, cost-effective, complication-free surgical procedures to maximize patient satisfaction. Hospitals and payers must also carefully consider the financial aspects of their health care decisions in a competitive environment with increasing costs, limited resources, and diminishing reimbursement.

Given the multifactorial nature of patient satisfaction and the highly complex and competitive medical setting, it becomes apparent why patient expectations after TKA are not always met. Patients undergoing this procedure often have a multitude of preoperative physical and psychological challenges that are not entirely resolved after TKA. Patient expectations may be unrealistic; outcomes may be limited by other comorbidities or complications that occur in the perioperative period. Surgeons' portrayals of the operations and potential outcomes may be overzealous and exaggerated. The perception of the success of the operation by the surgeon and the patient may be discordant, with the surgeon being the more optimistic. Surgeons or manufacturers may tout the benefits of a specific implant/surgical approach/perioperative protocol to patients to gain a competitive advantage. However, in most of these cases there is scant evidence to support this position. Although the protocols for controlling pain after TKA have perhaps been the most successful recent innovation, residual pain often is interpreted as an ominous complaint by both the frustrated patients and exasperated surgeons. This adverse result is seen more frequently in certain patient cohorts, such as workers' compensation cases and patients with underlying depression.[70,71] All of the concerns discussed earlier are currently being played out in an environment in which doctors, hospitals, and payers are being rated by patients online, with little to no recourse for rebuttal. How can this conundrum be solved to everyone's satisfaction? Table 2 summarizes important recommendations to improve TKA outcomes.

First, doctors and patients must engage in an open discussion about the surgical procedure, including indications, options, potential outcomes, and risk of complications. Both parties must be frank about their expectations and deliverables. All viable conservative measures should be exhausted before consideration of surgery. The surgeon should be cognizant of the physical demands of the patient's work and leisure activities, and together the surgeon and patient should decide whether TKA will live up to or fall short of their expectations. In particular, the possibility of unexplained residual pain should be discussed, despite what seems to be a clinically and radiographically sound reconstruction in the surgeon's eyes.[72,73] This discrepancy between what the surgeon thinks of as being a successful operation and the patient's expectations may lead to litigation.[74] Information regarding what to expect after TKA should be clearly stated preoperatively and inflated expectations should be mitigated to avoid frustration postoperatively.

Second, patients should be medically and psychologically prepared to undergo the operation and have sufficient resources and ancillary support to help ensure a successful outcome.[75] Optimization of medical, dental, and psychological health before surgery helps to mitigate perioperative complications. Unresolved issues related to finances, aftercare, housing, and work and family obligations place undue stress on the patient. Even the simple task of getting to and from the physical therapist's office may pose a challenge in an elderly patient with limited social supports.

Third, the surgical team, allied personnel, and the hospital should be focused on the delivery of patient-centered, high-quality, efficient, and

Table 2
Critical recommendations for better outcomes in total knee arthroplasty

General Recommendations	Details
Open discussion about the procedure preoperatively	Be frank and discuss conservative measures Have a complete knowledge of the patient's activities (work and leisure) Clearly state the expectations Convey the possibility of unexplained residual pain after the procedure
Preoperative preparation	Psychologically prepare the patient, counseling classes Optimization of medical comorbidities Help solve social issues
The medical team	Must be patient centered and offer high-quality services Use of validated protocols with flexibility to meet each patient's needs Remind the patient of the timeline for achievement of goals
After the procedure	Actively engage patients in their care Recognize successful steps and encourage the patient Do not underestimate complications and treat them actively
Associated actors (payers, medical societies)	Establish a tight collaboration and provide patients with understandable information Avoid costly and time-consuming, unnecessary treatments

cost-effective services. Preoperative counseling classes or information to better prepare patients for their operations have shown some success.[75] Specialized high-volume surgical teams, wards, or hospitals that can provide high-quality care consistently using validated protocols have also been shown to be useful, and provide clear benchmarks and timelines for achievement of specific goals. Some standardization of protocols is inevitable but sufficient flexibility must exist to recognize each patient's individual needs.

Fourth, patients must be highly engaged in their care and participate actively to help ensure a successful outcome. A patient's success highlights the success of the whole team and institution. Complications and adverse outcomes may in part be caused by a lack of compliance; for example, with uncontrolled diabetes, poor smoking habits, or missed physical therapy appointments. The burden of preoperative comorbidities has been evaluated in many studies. From a Danish registry, Glassou and colleagues[76] showed that current patients bear more comorbidities than their counterparts 15 years ago. Preexisting comorbidities before surgery are associated with lower scores for physical functioning and quality of life.[77–80] Therefore, optimizing patient comorbidities before proceeding to surgery is critical in order to obtain better outcomes.

Fifth, payers should remain highly collaborative in helping to establish evidence-based protocols to optimize outcome after TKA. Treatments that are not substantiated should be reevaluated and discontinued, or perhaps offered as an extra option, the cost of which is borne by the patient.

In addition, medical societies and local or national registries can help determine which procedures/implants/perioperative protocols are associated with the best outcomes and actively promote these activities.

In summary, it can be clearly seen that a variety of elements contribute to patients' satisfaction after TKA. The personality characteristics of the patient, surgical factors and the type of prosthesis chosen, perioperative control of pain and rehabilitation, and issues related to nursing and medical care all play important roles in patients' ratings of how pleased they are with the operative procedure. In many cases, the factors that affect the patient's satisfaction are seemingly contradictory or not within the surgeon's direct sphere of control. Moreover, the exact pathway to achieving patient satisfaction is similarly unclear.

Ultimately, although patient satisfaction is important, it should not be the definitive factor when evaluating the outcome of surgical procedures and patient care. Given the multifactorial nature of patient satisfaction, institutions should be wary of making surgeons bear the burden of the patients' pleasure/displeasure with their surgical procedures. This practice erodes the doctor-patient relationship further and leads to so-called cherry picking of patients by surgeons. These issues may have even broader implications for the surgeons' referral bases and economic well-being, given the renewed emphasis on patient satisfaction as a measure for financial reimbursement and the current online publication of patients' comments.

REFERENCES

1. Peck BM, Ubel PA, Roter DL, et al. Do unmet expectations for specific tests, referrals, and new medications reduce patients' satisfaction? J Gen Intern Med 2004;19(11):1080–7.
2. Sequist TD, Schneider EC, Anastario M, et al. Quality monitoring of physicians: linking patients' experiences of care to clinical quality and outcomes. J Gen Intern Med 2008;23(11):1784–90.
3. Fenton JJ, Jerant AF, Bertakis KD, et al. The cost of satisfaction: a national study of patient satisfaction, health care utilization, expenditures, and mortality. Arch Intern Med 2012;172(5):405–11.
4. The problem with satisfied patients. The Atlantic: The Atlantic Media Company 2015.
5. Lee K, Goodman SB. Current state and future of joint replacements in the hip and knee. Expert Rev Med Devices 2008;5(3):383–93.
6. Kurtz S, Ong K, Lau E, et al. Projections of primary and revision hip and knee arthroplasty in the United States from 2005 to 2030. J Bone Joint Surg Am 2007;89(4):780–5.
7. Wylde V, Hewlett S, Learmonth ID, et al. Persistent pain after joint replacement: prevalence, sensory qualities, and postoperative determinants. Pain 2011;152(3):566–72.
8. Beswick AD, Wylde V, Gooberman-Hill R, et al. What proportion of patients report long-term pain after total hip or knee replacement for osteoarthritis? A systematic review of prospective studies in unselected patients. BMJ Open 2012;2(1): e000435.
9. Nashi N, Hong CC, Krishna L. Residual knee pain and functional outcome following total knee arthroplasty in osteoarthritic patients. Knee Surg Sports Traumatol Arthrosc 2014;23:1841–7.
10. Wylde V, Blom AW, Whitehouse SL, et al. Patient-reported outcomes after total hip and knee

arthroplasty: comparison of midterm results. J Arthroplasty 2009;24(2):210–6.

11. Schnurr C, Jarrous M, Gudden I, et al. Pre-operative arthritis severity as a predictor for total knee arthroplasty patients' satisfaction. Int Orthop 2013;37(7):1257–61.

12. Clement ND. Patient factors that influence the outcome of total knee replacement: a critical review of the literature. Orthopaedics 2013;1(2):11.

13. Clement ND, MacDonald D, Simpson AH, et al. Total knee replacement in patients with concomitant back pain results in a worse functional outcome and a lower rate of satisfaction. Bone Joint J 2013;95B(12):1632–9.

14. McLawhorn AS, Bjerke-Kroll BT, Blevins JL, et al. Patient-reported allergies are associated with poorer patient satisfaction and outcomes after lower extremity arthroplasty: a retrospective cohort study. J Arthroplasty 2015;30(7):1132–6.

15. Maratt JD, Lee YY, Lyman S, et al. Predictors of satisfaction following total knee arthroplasty. J Arthroplasty 2015;30(7):1142–5.

16. Dunbar MJ, Richardson G, Robertsson O. I can't get no satisfaction after my total knee replacement: rhymes and reasons. Bone Joint J 2013;95B(11 Suppl A):148–52.

17. Hamilton DF, Lane JV, Gaston P, et al. What determines patient satisfaction with surgery? A prospective cohort study of 4709 patients following total joint replacement. BMJ Open 2013;3(4) [pii: e002525].

18. Culliton SE, Bryant DM, Overend TJ, et al. The relationship between expectations and satisfaction in patients undergoing primary total knee arthroplasty. J Arthroplasty 2012;27(3):490–2.

19. Jones DL, Bhanegaonkar AJ, Billings AA, et al. Differences between actual and expected leisure activities after total knee arthroplasty for osteoarthritis. J Arthroplasty 2012;27(7):1289–96.

20. Vissers MM, de Groot IB, Reijman M, et al. Functional capacity and actual daily activity do not contribute to patient satisfaction after total knee arthroplasty. BMC Musculoskelet Disord 2010;11:121.

21. Sjoling M, Nordahl G, Olofsson N, et al. The impact of preoperative information on state anxiety, postoperative pain and satisfaction with pain management. Patient Educ Couns 2003;51(2):169–76.

22. Matsuda S, Kawahara S, Okazaki K, et al. Postoperative alignment and ROM affect patient satisfaction after TKA. Clin Orthop Relat Res 2013;471(1):127–33.

23. Von Keudell A, Sodha S, Collins J, et al. Patient satisfaction after primary total and unicompartmental knee arthroplasty: an age-dependent analysis. Knee 2014;21(1):180–4.

24. Longo UG, Loppini M, Trovato U, et al. No difference between unicompartmental versus total knee arthroplasty for the management of medial osteoarthritis of the knee in the same patient: a systematic review and pooling data analysis. Br Med Bull 2015;114(1):65–73.

25. Jacobs CA, Christensen CP, Karthikeyan T. Patient and intraoperative factors influencing satisfaction two to five years after primary total knee arthroplasty. J Arthroplasty 2014;29(8):1576–9.

26. Costa CR, Johnson AJ, Harwin SF, et al. Critical review of minimally invasive approaches in knee arthroplasty. J Knee Surg 2013;26(1):41–50.

27. Cheng J, Liu J, Shi Z, et al. Interleukin-4 inhibits RANKL-induced NFATc1 expression via STAT6: a novel mechanism mediating its blockade of osteoclastogenesis. J Cell Biochem 2011;112(11):3385–92.

28. Bonutti PM, Zywiel MG, Ulrich SD, et al. A comparison of subvastus and midvastus approaches in minimally invasive total knee arthroplasty. J Bone Joint Surg Am 2010;92(3):575–82.

29. Nestor BJ, Toulson CE, Backus SI, et al. Mini-midvastus vs standard medial parapatellar approach: a prospective, randomized, double-blinded study in patients undergoing bilateral total knee arthroplasty. J Arthroplasty 2010;25(6 Suppl):5–11, 11.e1.

30. Xu SZ, Lin XJ, Tong X, et al. Minimally invasive midvastus versus standard parapatellar approach in total knee arthroplasty: a meta-analysis of randomized controlled trials. PLoS One 2014;9(5):e95311.

31. Gandhi R, de Beer J, Petruccelli D, et al. Does patient perception of alignment affect total knee arthroplasty outcome? Can J Surg 2007;50(3):181–6.

32. Rowe PJ, Myles CM, Walker C, et al. Knee joint kinematics in gait and other functional activities measured using flexible electrogoniometry: how much knee motion is sufficient for normal daily life? Gait Posture 2000;12(2):143–55.

33. Ritter MA, Lutgring JD, Davis KE, et al. The effect of postoperative range of motion on functional activities after posterior cruciate-retaining total knee arthroplasty. J Bone Joint Surg Am 2008;90(4):777–84.

34. Du H, Tang H, Gu JM, et al. Patient satisfaction after posterior-stabilized total knee arthroplasty: a functional specific analysis. Knee 2014;21(4):866–70.

35. Narayan K, Thomas G, Kumar R. Is extreme flexion of the knee after total knee replacement a prerequisite for patient satisfaction? Int Orthop 2009;33(3):671–4.

36. Devers BN, Conditt MA, Jamieson ML, et al. Does greater knee flexion increase patient function and

satisfaction after total knee arthroplasty? J Arthroplasty 2011;26(2):178–86.

37. Argenson JN, Parratte S, Ashour A, et al. Patient-reported outcome correlates with knee function after a single-design mobile-bearing TKA. Clin Orthop Relat Res 2008;466(11):2669–76.

38. Thomsen MG, Husted H, Otte KS, et al. Do patients care about higher flexion in total knee arthroplasty? A randomized, controlled, double-blinded trial. BMC Musculoskelet Disord 2013;14:127.

39. Boese CK, Gallo TJ, Plantikow CJ. Range of motion and patient satisfaction with traditional and high-flexion rotating-platform knees. Iowa Orthop J 2011;31:73–7.

40. Guild GN 3rd, Labib SA. Clinical outcomes in high flexion total knee arthroplasty were not superior to standard posterior stabilized total knee arthroplasty. A multicenter, prospective, randomized study. J Arthroplasty 2014;29(3):530–4.

41. Dennis DA, Heekin RD, Clark CR, et al. Effect of implant design on knee flexion. J Arthroplasty 2013;28(3):429–38.

42. Yun XD, Yin XL, Jiang J, et al. Local infiltration analgesia versus femoral nerve block in total knee arthroplasty: a meta-analysis. Orthop Traumatol Surg Res 2015;101:565–9.

43. Xu J, Chen XM, Ma CK, et al. Peripheral nerve blocks for postoperative pain after major knee surgery. Cochrane Database Syst Rev 2014;(12):CD010937.

44. Chan EY, Fransen M, Parker DA, et al. Femoral nerve blocks for acute postoperative pain after knee replacement surgery. Cochrane Database Syst Rev 2014;(5):CD009941.

45. Wang C, Cai XZ, Yan SG. Comparison of periarticular multimodal drug injection and femoral nerve block for postoperative pain management in total knee arthroplasty: a systematic review and meta-analysis. J Arthroplasty 2015;30(7):1281–6.

46. Buvanendran A, Kroin JS, Tuman KJ, et al. Effects of perioperative administration of a selective cyclooxygenase 2 inhibitor on pain management and recovery of function after knee replacement: a randomized controlled trial. JAMA 2003;290(18):2411–8.

47. Fischer HB, Simanski CJ, Sharp C, et al. A procedure-specific systematic review and consensus recommendations for postoperative analgesia following total knee arthroplasty. Anaesthesia 2008;63(10):1105–23.

48. Milani P, Castelli P, Sola M, et al. Multimodal analgesia in total knee arthroplasty: a randomized, double-blind, controlled trial on additional efficacy of periarticular anesthesia. J Arthroplasty 2015;30(11):2038–42.

49. Chang CB, Cho WS. Pain management protocols, peri-operative pain and patient satisfaction after total knee replacement: a multicentre study. J Bone Joint Surg Br 2012;94(11):1511–6.

50. Franklin PD, Karbassi JA, Li W, et al. Reduction in narcotic use after primary total knee arthroplasty and association with patient pain relief and satisfaction. J Arthroplasty 2010;25(6 Suppl):12–6.

51. Baker PN, van der Meulen JH, Lewsey J, et al, National Joint Registry for England and Wales. The role of pain and function in determining patient satisfaction after total knee replacement. Data from the National Joint Registry for England and Wales. J Bone Joint Surg Br 2007;89(7):893–900.

52. Pozzi F, Snyder-Mackler L, Zeni J. Physical exercise after knee arthroplasty: a systematic review of controlled trials. Eur J Phys Rehabil Med 2013;49(6):877–92.

53. Minns Lowe CJ, Barker KL, Dewey M, et al. Effectiveness of physiotherapy exercise after knee arthroplasty for osteoarthritis: systematic review and meta-analysis of randomised controlled trials. BMJ 2007;335(7624):812.

54. Bade MJ, Stevens-Lapsley JE. Restoration of physical function in patients following total knee arthroplasty: an update on rehabilitation practices. Curr Opin Rheumatol 2012;24(2):208–14.

55. Wang T-J, Chang C-F, Lou M-F, et al. Biofeedback relaxation for pain associated with continuous passive motion in Taiwanese patients after total knee arthroplasty. Res Nurs Health 2015;38(1):39–50.

56. Joshi RN, White PB, Murray-Weir M, et al. Prospective randomized trial of the efficacy of continuous passive motion post total knee arthroplasty: experience of the hospital for special surgery. J Arthroplasty 2015;30:2364–9.

57. Herbold JA, Bonistall K, Blackburn M, et al. Randomized controlled trial of the effectiveness of continuous passive motion after total knee replacement. Arch Phys Med Rehabil 2014;95(7):1240–5.

58. Baumann C, Rat AC, Osnowycz G, et al. Satisfaction with care after total hip or knee replacement predicts self-perceived health status after surgery. BMC Musculoskelet Disord 2009;10:150.

59. Webster F, Bremner S, Katz J, et al. Patients' perceptions of joint replacement care in a changing healthcare system: a qualitative study. Healthc Policy 2014;9(3):55–66.

60. Bovonratwet P, Webb ML, Ondeck NT, et al. Definitional differences of 'outpatient' versus 'inpatient' THA and TKA can affect study outcomes. Clin Orthop Relat Res 2017. [Epub ahead of print].

61. Bovonratwet P, Ondeck NT, Nelson SJ, et al. Comparison of outpatient vs inpatient total knee arthroplasty: an ACS-NSQIP analysis. J Arthroplasty 2017;32:1773–8.

62. Pollock M, Somerville L, Firth A, et al. Outpatient total hip arthroplasty, total knee arthroplasty, and

unicompartmental knee arthroplasty: a systematic review of the literature. JBJS Rev 2016;4(12) [pii: 01874474-201612000-00004].

63. Lovecchio F, Alvi H, Sahota S, et al. Is outpatient arthroplasty as safe as fast-track inpatient arthroplasty? A propensity score matched analysis. J Arthroplasty 2016;31(9 Suppl):197–201.

64. Kolisek FR, McGrath MS, Jessup NM, et al. Comparison of outpatient versus inpatient total knee arthroplasty. Clin Orthop Relat Res 2009;467(6): 1438–42.

65. Grissom SP, Dunagan L. Improved satisfaction during inpatient rehabilitation after hip and knee arthroplasty: a retrospective analysis. Am J Phys Med Rehabil 2001;80(11):798–803.

66. Ali A, Sundberg M, Robertsson O, et al. Dissatisfied patients after total knee arthroplasty: a registry study involving 114 patients with 8–13 years of follow-up. Acta Orthop 2014;85(3):229–33.

67. Kumar M, Battepathi P, Bangalore P. Expectation fulfilment and satisfaction in total knee arthroplasty patients using the 'PROFEX' questionnaire. Orthop Traumatol Surg Res 2015;101(3):325–30.

68. Carr-Hill RA. The measurement of patient satisfaction. J Public Health Med 1992;14(3):236–49.

69. Kurtz SM, Ong KL, Lau E, et al. Impact of the economic downturn on total joint replacement demand in the United States: updated projections to 2021. J Bone Joint Surg Am 2014;96(8): 624–30.

70. Mont MA, Mayerson JA, Krackow KA, et al. Total knee arthroplasty in patients receiving workers' compensation. J Bone Joint Surg Am 1998;80(9): 1285–90.

71. Saleh K, Nelson C, Kassim R, et al. Total knee arthroplasty in patients on workers' compensation: a matched cohort study with an average follow-up of 4.5 years. J Arthroplasty 2004;19(3):310–2.

72. Manning BT, Lewis N, Tzeng TH, et al. Diagnosis and management of extra-articular causes of pain after total knee arthroplasty. Instr Course Lect 2015;64:381–8.

73. Potty AG, Tzeng TH, Sams JD, et al. Diagnosis and management of intra-articular causes of pain after total knee arthroplasty. Instr Course Lect 2015;64: 389–401.

74. Gibon E, Farman T, Marmor S. Knee arthroplasty and lawsuits: the experience in France. Knee Surg Sports Traumatol Arthrosc 2014;23:3723–8.

75. Cook JR, Warren M, Ganley KJ, et al. A comprehensive joint replacement program for total knee arthroplasty: a descriptive study. BMC Musculoskelet Disord 2008;9:154.

76. Glassou EN, Pedersen AB, Hansen TB. Is decreasing mortality in total hip and knee arthroplasty patients dependent on patients' comorbidity? Acta Orthop 2017;1–6.

77. Elmallah RDK, Cherian JJ, Robinson K, et al. The effect of comorbidities on outcomes following total knee arthroplasty. J Knee Surg 2015;28(5):411–6.

78. Lizaur-Utrilla A, Gonzalez-Parreño S, Miralles-Muñoz FA, et al. Patient-related predictors of treatment failure after primary total knee arthroplasty for osteoarthritis. J Arthroplasty 2014;29(11):2095–9.

79. Desmeules F, Dionne CE, Belzile EL, et al. Determinants of pain, functional limitations and health-related quality of life six months after total knee arthroplasty: results from a prospective cohort study. BMC Sports Sci Med Rehabil 2013;5:2.

80. Wylde V, Dieppe P, Hewlett S, et al. Total knee replacement: is it really an effective procedure for all? Knee 2007;14(6):417–23.

Trauma

The Effect of Opioids, Alcohol, and Nonsteroidal Anti-inflammatory Drugs on Fracture Union

Christopher J. Richards, MD, MS[a,*],
Kenneth W. Graf Jr, MD[b], Rakesh P. Mashru, MD[b]

KEYWORDS

- Fracture • Nonunion • Opioids • Alcohol • NSAIDs

KEY POINTS

- Retrospective clinical studies show a negative correlation between opioids and fracture healing, but there is no study that can determine direct causality.
- Animal models suggest that alcohol has an inhibitory effect on osteoblast proliferation and leads to a detrimental effect on fracture healing.
- Animal models have suggested that NSAIDs are a risk factor for nonunion; however, retrospective studies on human fracture data have failed to definitively link NSAIDs and nonunion.
- There are limited data to allow for clinical guidelines regarding opioids, alcohol, and NSAIDs on fracture union; rather, the prescribing physician should be cognizant of the potential effects.

INTRODUCTION

Fracture union is a complex process that is intimately related to the biologic and mechanical environments at the fracture site. Improper fracture fixation ranging from undersized intramedullary nails to overstiffened plate constructs can create an unfavorable mechanical environment for fracture union (**Fig. 1** and **Fig. 2**). In the biologic environment, a multitude of cells and molecules are found at fracture sites within hours, and work to provide a framework for fracture repair. There are multiple inflammatory cells found at fracture sites within hours of the injury, and play an influential role in hematoma formation and the early stages of fracture healing within the first 5 days.[1] A multitude of factors influencing fracture union have been suggested including nutritional status; endocrine disorders; smoking; fracture location; fracture energy; fracture pattern; and medications, including steroids, chemotherapy agents, and nonsteroidal anti-inflammatory drugs (NSAIDs).[1] External factors influencing fracture union have come under increasing scrutiny in efforts to reduce the rates of nonunion or delayed union. Particularly, patient nutritional status and smoking status have proven to be influential in fracture healing as a result of altering the molecular environment at the fracture site.[1] Several medications have also come under consideration for their theoretic ability to alter the early inflammatory pathway and the later molecular environment involved in the formation of new bone. For

---

Disclosure Statement: None of the authors have any disclosures.
[a] Department of Orthopaedic Surgery, Cooper University Hospital, 3 Cooper Plaza, Camden, NJ 08103, USA;
[b] Department of Orthopaedic Surgery, Cooper Medical School of Rowan University, 401 South Broadway, Camden, NJ 08103, USA
* Corresponding author.
E-mail address: Richards-christopher@cooperhealth.edu

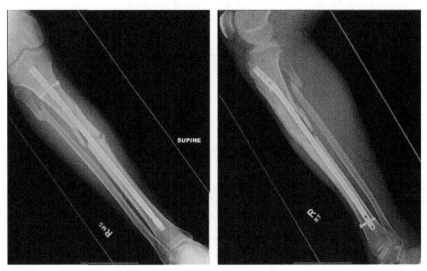

Fig. 1. Atrophic nonunion resulting from an undersized tibial nail.

example, there is a theoretic risk of chronic corticosteroid use leading to impaired fracture union because of the inhibition of osteogenic differentiation of mesenchymal stem cells, but this has not been proven in clinical studies.[1]

Although there is no standard definition of nonunion, it is generally accepted that nonunion is defined as a lack of complete bone healing within a specified time frame, typically between 6 and 9 months.[1] Nonunion is a known complication of the operative and nonoperative management of fractures. The rate of fracture nonunion has been estimated to be between 5% and 10%.[2] The effects of fracture nonunion are

detrimental to the patient and the health care system. Some estimates of tibial shaft nonunions suggest that the median health care cost of nonunion versus union was more than two times greater, despite nonunions representing only 12% of tibial fractures overall.[3] With the increasing focus on patient outcomes and the awareness of external factors that influence fracture union, surgeon- and patient-controlled variables are being increasingly studied. Although smoking is generally accepted as detrimental to fracture healing, a less discussed patient factor is alcohol. Some studies demonstrate an association between alcohol use and impaired

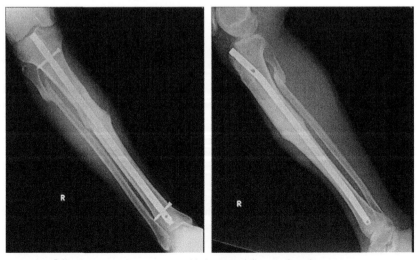

Fig. 2. Fracture union following nonunion surgery with intramedullary nail exchange.

fracture healing, with animal studies suggesting that it is a result of the inhibition of osteoblast proliferation.[4–19]

Specific surgeon-controlled factors are pain-control modalities following operative and nonoperative fracture care. NSAIDs and opioids are two widely used medications to help with pain control in the acute postfracture setting. NSAIDs are commonly used pain medications that target the inflammatory cascade. Because normal fracture healing involves an early inflammatory response, theoretically NSAIDs could interfere with normal fracture healing biology, resulting in a delayed union or a nonunion. Numerous animal models have suggested that NSAIDs can play a role in fracture healing; however, clinical studies have resulted in conflicting recommendations regarding the use of NSAIDs with fractures.[20–37] Opioids are also frequently prescribed medications by orthopedic physicians and there has been some recent suggestion of opioids influencing fracture union. Although literature is limited on the effect of opioids on fracture union, with no study able to demonstrate causality, there is some suggestion in animal studies and retrospective clinical studies of a negative influence on fracture union.[2,3,22,38–40] Pain control is an important consideration of patient care, and the treating physicians should be aware of the potential negative side effects of the medications that they are prescribing. To date, there are no defined clinical recommendations regarding a pain management regimen in the setting of fracture with respect to the effects on fracture union. This article reviews the current literature to examine the effects of opioids, alcohol, and NSAIDs on fracture union (Box 1, Box 2, and Box 3 for a summary of key points for each section).

METHODS OF LITERATURE REVIEW

A PubMed search was performed to review the current literature regarding fracture union. The search was generated with several combinations of multiple keywords: fracture, union, malunion, heal, healing, opioid, alcohol, and NSAIDs. The following search was used: fracture AND (union OR malunion OR nonunion OR heal OR healing) and (opioid OR alcohol OR NSAIDs). Additionally, the following MeSH terms were used: Fracture Healing [MeSH], Fractures, ununited [MeSH], and Fractures, malunited [MeSH].

The search was limited to peer-reviewed journal articles in the English language published between January 2000 and February 2017. The authors evaluated each article to determine relevance. The reference lists of selected articles were examined for additional relevant articles. Ultimately, the search yielded 40 articles that were deemed relevant.

OPIOIDS AND FRACTURE UNION

Opioids are a mainstay of pain management in the perioperative period among all surgical specialties. Orthopedic patients are no exception, with approximately 80% of fracture patients receiving opioids for analgesia.[41] Given the propensity for orthopedic patients to receive opioids while inpatient and after hospital discharge, an understanding of their effect on fracture healing is absolutely crucial.

The literature focusing on opioids and their effect on fracture union is primarily comprised of animal fracture models and retrospective reviews of human fracture data. The general consensus among the animal fracture models is that opioids impair fracture healing. Chrastil and colleagues[38] demonstrated this with a femoral osteotomy model with rats where one study group received saline and one study group received morphine for 8 weeks. At the conclusion of the study, the rats exposed to morphine demonstrated a decreased rate of fracture callus maturation, ultimately resulting in a weaker fracture callus. The control group fracture callus volume at 8 weeks was lower than that of the morphine-exposed group, suggesting that morphine possibly inhibited fracture callus remodeling and resorption.[38] Following this, Chrastil and colleagues[39] then used their femoral osteotomy rat model to investigate

---

Box 1
Summary of key points for opioids and fracture union

- Animal models demonstrate a negative impact of opioids on fracture healing
- Human data are retrospective and show an association of opioids negatively affecting fracture healing, but there is no study that can determine direct causality
- Further research must be conducted on this topic

> **Box 2**
> **Summary of key points for alcohol and fracture union**
>
> - Alcohol is commonly known as a risk factor for fracture, but its role in the healing of these fractures has been less commonly discussed
> - Animal models suggest an inhibition of osteoblast proliferation and function leads to alcohol's detrimental effect on fracture healing; the mechanism of this not entirely elucidated, but several pathways involving Wnt/β-catenin, transforming growth factor-β1, and mesenchymal stem cell function have been identified
> - Physicians must be cognizant of alcohol use in their patients postoperatively because this can drastically affect their recovery

whether opioid-induced androgen deficiency could be responsible for the decreased rate of callus maturation, but the authors failed to support this hypothesis. Chrastil and colleagues[39] ultimately proposed that opioids' inhibition of fracture callus maturation could be multifactorial, because opioids affect nearly every hypothalamic-pituitary-peripheral gland axis in the human body.

Given the well-documented negative effect of opioids on fracture healing, it is reasonable to consider that antagonism of these same receptors could actually promote fracture healing. Petrizzi and colleagues[40] used a common opioid antagonist, naloxone, and a bicortical drill hole model in a group of sheep to investigate this concept further. The researchers drilled a bicortical hole in the left metacarpus in a group of sheep and divided the sheep into various study groups. Each group received saline, calcium gluconate, naloxone, or both naloxone and calcium gluconate for 4 weeks. Monitoring bone healing radiographically and histologically, the group determined there was significantly faster healing in the naloxone and naloxone plus calcium gluconate group in comparison with the control group and calcium gluconate group.[40] The naloxone plus calcium gluconate group also healed significantly faster the naloxone only group. The authors concluded that naloxone enhances mineralization and remodeling in the

fracture callus of sheep, and this effect is potentiated by the concurrent administration of calcium gluconate.[40] These results suggest naloxone could be used as a potential pharmacologic treatment of nonunion, or prophylaxis for patients where this is of considerable risk.

The human studies investigating the effect of opioids on fracture healing are retrospective chart reviews examining different factors that influence fracture healing. Although the animal models clearly suggest a direct negative impact of opioids on fracture healing, the human data are not as forthright. Although Bhattacharyya and colleagues[22] calculated an odds ratio of 2.7 for opioid use and nonunion of humeral shaft fractures, the authors actually suggest this to be protopathic bias, where the use of analgesic medication is essentially a marker for a painful nonhealing fracture. More recently, large retrospective reviews by Antonova and colleagues[3] and Zura and colleagues[2] examining factors affecting fracture nonunion demonstrated a propensity for nonunion in the patients using opioids for pain management, but given the retrospective nature of these studies, causality cannot be further investigated. By and large, the human data on the effect of opioids on fracture healing are lacking, and further research in this field is necessary to properly guide perioperative analgesia in these patients.

> **Box 3**
> **Summary of key points for NSAIDs and fracture union**
>
> - Cyclooxygenase-2 is closely involved in fracture repair and inhibition of this enzyme leads to impaired fracture healing in animal models
> - Retrospective reviews of human fracture data are inconclusive as to whether there is an association with NSAIDs and fracture nonunion
> - Most authors agree that a short duration of NSAID use is safe in fracture patients as long as the patients have no other risk factors for nonunion

ALCOHOL AND FRACTURE UNION

Individuals who abuse alcohol are four times more likely to suffer a fracture than their age-matched control subjects, and 25% to 40% of orthopedic trauma patients are intoxicated at the time of admission.[42,43] Although alcohol is well known as a cause of poor bone health and therefore serves as a risk factor for orthopedic injuries, the effect of alcohol on the healing of these injuries is less commonly addressed. Despite its lack of recognition as a significant cause of impaired fracture healing, alcohol abuse has been cited as one of the most predictive factors for nonunion, particularly for younger patients with femoral neck fractures.[8]

Animal models constitute most studies investigating the effects of alcohol and fracture healing, and the findings of these models have been consistent. Brown and colleagues[4] used a distraction osteogenesis model to investigate alcohol and fracture healing. Distraction osteogenesis is a clinical technique where an osteotomy is performed and an external fixator is applied to slowly separate the two pieces of bone.[4] Separation leads to rapid bone formation in the slowly expanding gap, and thus, this can be used as a model for fracture healing. The study was multifaceted and had several subgroups, each using an intragastric cannula to provide the experimental rats with chronic alcohol exposure and the control rats with a control liquid diet. The subgroups undergoing distraction osteogenesis either received 2 weeks of control diet or alcohol before beginning distraction osteogenesis, followed by 16 more days of control diet or alcohol while the external fixator slowly distracted the two pieces of the tibia. The results showed decreased intramembranous bone formation and the authors attributed this primarily to decreased osteoblast proliferation and function because this had been demonstrated in several studies prior.[4,44–46]

Chakkalakal and colleagues[6] used a rat model to perform several studies surrounding this topic. In their initial study, the authors performed bilateral fibular osteotomies and bridged the gap with demineralized bone matrix. The animals were divided into four groups: Group A received an alcohol liquid diet constituting 36% of total caloric intake; Group B served as a control group and received 36% maltodextrin instead of alcohol; Group C was given a standard AIN-93M rodent diet, which is an open formula diet published by the American Institute of Nutrition; and Group D was initially given the alcohol liquid diet but then switched to the AIN-93M rodent diet postinjury. The animals were acclimated to their diet for 6 weeks before injury, and the experiment continued for 7 weeks postinjury. The authors saw that Group A had impaired bone healing compared with the other groups, and Group D showed comparable bone healing to Group C.[6] Naturally, this difference in fracture healing was attributed to the alcohol exposure. However, the authors saw a significant difference in weight gain between Groups A and B and Groups C and D, and considered that weight gain could be a confounding variable.

They repeated a similar experiment several years later using varying levels of alcohol intake (36% of total calories deemed "high ethanol consumption" and 26% of total calories deemed "moderate ethanol consumption") and additional nutritional control groups for comparison.[47] The study produced similar results, showcasing impaired healing in the high-ethanol consumption group, normal healing in the moderate ethanol consumption group, and restoration of normal bone healing in the group where alcohol was removed immediately postinjury.[47] The authors concluded that the change in bone healing was caused by the alcohol exposure and not the reduced food intake in the alcohol-exposed rats. The underlying mechanism of this phenomenon still remains to be fully elucidated, but the authors suggest the impaired osteoblast proliferation and function leads to a disruption in the formation of ossifiable matrix and/or its subsequent mineralization, ultimately resulting in weaker fracture callus formation.[47] Other studies have suggested that impaired osteoblastic activity leads to increased activity of fibroblasts and/or chondroblasts, additionally contributing to a weaker repair tissue composed of fibrous tissue and/or cartilage.[4,9] Whether the impaired osteoblastic activity lies in direct inhibition of osteoblastic proliferation or their differentiation from mesenchymal stem cells at the site of injury still remains in question.[5]

Trevisiol and colleagues[18] did not use an animal fracture model, but instead studied osteoinduction by subcutaneously implanting four pieces of demineralized allogeneic bone matrix into rats. Two pieces were placed in the thorax and two more in the abdomen, the experimental group was exposed to a diet composed of 35% ethanol for 6 weeks, and then the implanted bone was removed for analysis. The authors discovered that the total amount of bone formed in the experimental group compared with the control group was decreased, specifically with a decrease in connectivity density (the amount of connections between trabeculae), trabecular number, and trabecular thickness and an increase in the structural model index (which is a characterization score of the trabecular geometry). Taken together, these findings illustrate the effects of decreased osteoblast function and number.[18]

The specifics surrounding the dysfunction of osteoblasts as a result of ethanol exposure have been studied in vitro rather extensively. Torricelli and colleagues[17] subjected osteoblasts to ethanol in vitro, and then seeded them in immediate contact with a pure titanium orthopedic implant. The osteoblasts exposed to ethanol had a decrease in production of various extracellular matrix proteins, such as type 1 collagen, osteocalcin, and alkaline phosphatase (ALP).[10,17] The authors also noted a disruption in local regulatory molecules involved in fracture repair, such that transforming growth factor (TGF)-β1 was decreased, whereas tumor necrosis factor-α and interleukin-6 levels were increased.[17]

Following the numerous studies suggesting alcohol-induced osteoblastic dysfunction was the culprit of impaired fracture healing, several studies furthered this knowledge by looking at specific molecular pathways involved in bone healing. Specifically, these studies looked at the canonical Wnt/β-catenin pathway. This pathway has been well described as an integral component of normal fracture healing because it involves the differentiation of mesenchymal stem cells into osteoblasts and chondroblasts.[48–50] Volkmer and colleagues,[19] Lauing and colleagues,[12] and Roper and colleagues[15] each used animal models to demonstrate that alcohol disrupts Wnt/β-catenin signaling, ultimately leading to impaired fracture repair.

It has been hypothesized previously that alcohol generates reactive oxygen species, and the increased oxidative stress induces transcription of Forkhead Box O (FoxO) genes.[51–53] When FoxO genes are transcribed, β-catenin then binds to FoxO proteins instead of the appropriate transcription factors in the Wnt pathway, leading to overall decreased Wnt/β-catenin pathway activity.[51,52] Volkmer and colleagues[19] and Roper and colleagues[15] both used an additional experimental group where the rats received alcohol and N-acetylcysteine (NAC), a well-known antioxidant. The addition of NAC attenuated the negative effect of ethanol on fracture repair, and improved the biomechanical strength of the fracture callus to

a level comparable with that of the control group. NAC is believed to have stopped the formation of reactive oxygen species and therefore, blunted the negative effect of alcohol on Wnt/β-catenin pathway activity, ultimately leading to normal fracture healing. These findings not only support the hypothesis that alcohol ingestion generates oxidative stress and disrupts Wnt/β-catenin signaling, but also suggest a more clinical application of NAC as a potential therapeutic intervention for orthopedic trauma patients at risk for nonunion.

Other potential interventions to effectively curtail alcohol's deleterious effects on fracture healing have been studied. Prior studies have shown that β-catenin can be targeted for degradation by glycogen synthase kinase 3 beta, a molecule that is upregulated by alcohol exposure. On the contrary, lithium chloride is an inhibitor of that kinase and prevents its action on β-catenin.[48,54] Lauing and colleagues[13] subjected rats to midshaft tibial fractures, exposed one group to saline and two experimental groups to binge alcohol use, and concurrently administered lithium chloride to one of those ethanol-exposed groups. Lithium chloride effectively blunted alcohol's negative effect by normalizing activated glycogen synthase kinase 3 beta levels to that of the control group, ultimately restoring endochondral ossification and fracture callus formation in the ethanol plus lithium chloride group.[13]

Mesenchymal stem cells play a key role in fracture repair. Obermeyer and colleagues[14] sought to further study the role of mesenchymal stem cells in fracture healing, specifically the role of these cells as a potential therapeutic technique in alcohol-related fracture nonunions. The authors used a binge drinking model in mice where they exposed the mice to alcohol for 3 days followed by 4 days of sobriety for a period of 2 weeks, and then subjected the mice to a midshaft tibial fracture while intoxicated. Mesenchymal stem cells harvested from the bone marrow of transgenic green fluorescent protein–expressing mice were administered intravenously at 24 hours postinjury, and their migration to the site of injury was monitored via fluorescence imaging. The study showed these cells were capable of migrating to the fracture site and contributing to fracture healing, such that the mechanical, histologic, and microcomputed tomography evidence of fracture healing was normalized to that of the control group exposed to saline.[14] Thus, systemic administration of mesenchymal stem cells represents a possible noninvasive therapeutic approach to prevention and treatment of nonunions.

The exact pathway through which mesenchymal stem cells exert their effect on fracture healing has not been entirely made clear, but Driver and colleagues[7] investigated a specific pathway involving TGF-β1 and osteopontin. It has been previously shown that mesenchymal stem cells release TGF-β1 via induction by osteopontin.[55] The osteopontin-induced TGF-β1 release is mediated by a transcription factor known as myeloid zinc finger 1 (MZF1), because MZF1 activates the TGF-β1 promoter. The authors studied the effects of ethanol exposure on this pathway in vitro with isolated mesenchymal stem cells and in vivo with a mouse tibial fracture model. They determined that alcohol interferes with MZF1 activity, ultimately leading to decreased activity of the pathway overall and impaired fracture callus formation.[7] Further studies are required to better characterize this phenomenon and offer potential therapeutic targets.

The general consensus of the literature is that alcohol directly impacts bone healing via disruption of several signaling pathways crucial to bone formation. Several potential therapeutic targets have been identified thus far, and further characterization of these affected molecular signaling cascades will allow for more directed development of interventional strategies to combat nonunion in these high-risk patients.

NONSTEROIDAL ANTI-INFLAMMATORY DRUGS AND FRACTURE UNION

NSAIDs are a commonly used group of medications in orthopedic patients given their anti-inflammatory, antipyretic, and analgesic effects. NSAIDs exert these effects via inhibition of the cyclooxygenase (COX)-1 and COX-2 enzymes and the resultant decrease in synthesis of proinflammatory prostaglandins.[56] COX-1 is constitutively expressed in most cells throughout the body and is heavily involved in homeostatic physiologic processes. On the contrary, COX-2 is considered to be an enzyme that is induced by inflammation and its activity is influenced by the presence of other inflammatory molecules.[56] It is hypothesized that NSAIDs exert their desired therapeutic effects via inhibition of COX-2, and inhibition of COX-1 leads to the well-known side effects of these medications, such as those involving the gastrointestinal tract and kidneys.[56,57] However, a theoretic side effect that is not commonly discussed is impaired fracture healing.

Beck and colleagues[21] used an animal model to investigate the effect of NSAIDs on fracture healing. Rats were divided into four groups and subjected to a transverse osteotomy of the left proximal tibia followed by exposure to either (1) placebo, (2) tramadol, (3) diclofenac for 7 days followed by placebo for 14 days, or (4) diclofenac for 21 days. After the healing period of 21 days, the repaired bone was examined. The authors noted that both diclofenac groups exhibited impaired fracture healing when compared with the placebo and tramadol groups. The authors hypothesized that the negative effect of diclofenac must be exerted early in the healing phase, because one of the groups was only exposed to diclofenac for a total of 7 days yet still displayed impaired fracture healing.[21]

In the previously described study, diclofenac acted as a nonselective NSAID, inhibiting COX-1 and COX-2. However, newer NSAIDs have been developed that predominantly inhibit COX-2, and are known as "selective COX-2 inhibitors." They are generally regarded as having a more favorable side effect profile than nonselective NSAIDs given their lack of effect on COX-1 activity.[26] However, COX-2 is largely responsible for the production of prostaglandin E_2, a molecule that is produced by osteoblasts to promote bone formation.[25,31] Investigators hypothesized that it was the inhibition of COX-2 and resultant decreased prostaglandin E_2 synthesis that was primarily responsible for the impaired fracture healing seen with NSAID use.[58] Simon and colleagues[58] investigated this concept with a closed femur fracture model in rats treated with selective COX-2 inhibitors. The authors saw that celecoxib and rofecoxib impaired fracture healing and attributed this to their selective COX-2 inhibition. The group then confirmed their hypothesis by examining fracture healing in mice with targeted homozygous null mutations in either the Cox1 or Cox2 gene. Lack of a functional Cox2 gene led to impaired fracture healing, supporting the group's hypothesis that COX-2 activity is essential for fracture repair.[58,59]

A study by Daluiski and colleagues[24] further investigated COX-2 and its role in fracture healing by directly measuring expression of COX-2 in human samples of nonunion callous and healed fracture callous. The authors used expression profiling to measure the COX-2 levels in each of the samples and determined that the nonunion samples had a 13-fold decrease in local levels of COX-2 expression. Additionally, this study examined if COX-2 was necessary for bone morphogenetic protein–induced osteogenesis by treating human osteoprogenitor cell line Saos-2 cells with celecoxib or dimethylsulfoxide, an organic solvent that dissolves celecoxib, for 72 hours and measuring their ALP activity on exposure to bone morphogenetic protein. ALP is a particularly sensitive marker for osteogenesis, and the Saos-2 cells typically produce ALP in response to bone morphogenetic protein.[24] The authors saw that when the two groups of cells were exposed to bone morphogenetic protein, the cells treated with celecoxib showcased a significant and dose-dependent decrease in ALP activity compared with that of the control group. The group concluded that inhibition of COX-2 reduces the osteogenic potential of these cells, and that prostaglandin synthesis via COX-2 activity is required for bone morphogenetic–induced osteogenesis.[24]

After numerous studies showed that NSAIDs inhibited fracture repair, Gerstenfeld and colleagues[26] used a femur fracture model in rats to determine if the effects of NSAIDs on fracture healing were reversible after discontinuation of the drug. The authors exposed the experimental group animals to a nonselective NSAID, ketorolac, or a selective COX-2 inhibitor, valdecoxib, for either 7 or 21 days. The 7-day treatment did not produce significant differences in nonunion among the ketorolac, valdecoxib, or control groups, but the data did show that the 21-day treatment produced a significantly increased number of nonunions in the valdecoxib-exposed animals. However, with discontinuation of valdecoxib at 21 days, the difference in healing among the ketorolac, valdecoxib, and control groups disappeared by 35 days. The group concluded that COX-2 inhibition impairs fracture healing, but this is reversible after withdrawal of the offending agent.[26]

A common concern raised regarding these animal models is whether these data are applicable to humans. Although there have been numerous retrospective review articles analyzing human fracture healing and NSAID use, the data have been less than conclusive. One study by Giannoudis and colleagues[20] showed an association between diclofenac and ibuprofen use and nonunion of diaphyseal femur fractures (odds ratio, 10.74). Additionally, a study in 2014 focusing on nonunion of long-bone fractures demonstrated a two-fold-increased risk of nonunion in patients using NSAIDs after their injury.[35] Zura and colleagues[2] saw an increased risk of nonunion with patients taking both opioids and NSAIDs concurrently (odds ratio, 1.84). One study by Hernandez and colleagues[30] actually analyzed NSAID use before fracture and saw that NSAID use within 1 year before injury was associated with a two-fold increase in nonunion. However, this study did not look at recency, duration, or dosage of the NSAID used.

On the contrary, several studies have produced data showing no association between NSAIDs and impaired fracture healing. A study by Bhattacharyya and colleagues[22] claimed that the association of postoperative analgesic use and nonunions was protopathic bias and these patients were treating the pain of their unstable fractures. Interestingly, a meta-analysis by Dodwell and colleagues[29] analyzing the quality of studies and their results regarding NSAIDs and nonunion rates showed that lower-quality studies had higher reported odds ratios for nonunion with NSAID exposure. The study quality was determined via the Newcastle-Ottawa scale, and of note, when only high-quality studies were analyzed, there was no significant association between NSAID use and nonunion.[60] Furthermore, a study by DePeter and colleagues[37] showed no association between ibuprofen use and complications in the healing of various pediatric fractures.

One prospective study in human subjects by Park and colleagues[23] examined the use of ketorolac via patient controlled analgesia (PCA) in spinal fusion patients. The study consisted of 88 patients undergoing lumbar spinal fusion for spinal stenosis or spondylolisthesis. The patients were divided into two groups: one group received fentanyl and ketorolac intravenously via PCA postoperatively, and the other group received only fentanyl via PCA postoperatively. The authors saw a statistically significant difference in union rates among the two groups, with a relative risk of nonunion or incomplete union nearly six times higher (odds ratio, 5.64) in the ketorolac and fentanyl group. The group concluded that NSAIDs should be avoided in spinal fusion patients.[23]

Although it is clear that animal data strongly show that NSAID exposure is associated with nonunion, the human data are not as definitive. The general consensus among researchers and clinicians is that NSAIDs may inhibit fracture healing in humans to some extent, but a short duration of NSAID use after fracture is generally safe in patients who do not have other risk factors for nonunion.[27,28,31–34,36,61]

SUMMARY

Data in the current literature are limited to be able to define a causal relationship between opioids, alcohol, and NSAIDs and fracture nonunion. Although animal studies have suggested a negative effect of alcohol and NSAIDs on fracture union, retrospective clinical studies have failed to definitively reach a consensus and show a negative correlation. Retrospective clinical studies show a negative correlation between opioids and fracture healing, but there is no study that can determine direct causality. Further research is needed to define clinical guidelines regarding the use of opioids, alcohol, and NSAIDs in the setting of fracture, but treating physicians should be aware of the potential negative effects on fracture union.

ACKNOWLEDGMENTS

The authors thank Ryan D. DeAngelis for his significant contributions to this article.

REFERENCES

1. Court-Brown CM, Heckman JD, McQueen MM, et al. Rockwood and Green's fractures in adults. 8th edition. Philadelphia: Lippincott Williams & Wilkins; 2015. Available at: http://www.r2library.com.ezproxy.rowan.edu/resource/title/1451175310. Accessed March 10, 2017.

2. Zura R, Xiong Z, Einhorn T, et al. Epidemiology of fracture nonunion in 18 human bones. JAMA Surg 2016;151(11):e162775.

3. Antonova E, Le TK, Burge R, et al. Tibia shaft fractures: costly burden of nonunions. BMC Musculoskelet Disord 2013;14:42.

4. Brown EC, Perrien DS, Fletcher TW, et al. Skeletal toxicity associated with chronic ethanol exposure in a rat model using total enteral nutrition. J Pharmacol Exp Ther 2002;301(3):1132–8.

5. Chakkalakal DA. Alcohol-induced bone loss and deficient bone repair. Alcohol Clin Exp Res 2005; 29(12):2077–90.

6. Chakkalakal DA, Novak JR, Fritz ED, et al. Chronic ethanol consumption results in deficient bone repair in rats. Alcohol Alcohol 2002;37(1):13–20.

7. Driver J, Weber CE, Callaci JJ, et al. Alcohol inhibits osteopontin-dependent transforming growth factor-beta1 expression in human mesenchymal stem cells. J Biol Chem 2015;290(16):9959–73.

8. Duckworth AD, Bennet SJ, Aderinto J, et al. Fixation of intracapsular fractures of the femoral neck in young patients: risk factors for failure. J Bone Joint Surg Br 2011;93(6):811–6.

9. Elmali N, Ertem K, Ozen S, et al. Fracture healing and bone mass in rats fed on liquid diet containing ethanol. Alcohol Clin Exp Res 2002;26(4):509–13.

10. Fini M, Giavaresi G, Salamanna F, et al. Harmful lifestyles on orthopedic implantation surgery: a descriptive review on alcohol and tobacco use. J Bone Miner Metab 2011;29(6):633–44.

11. Gonzalez-Reimers E, Quintero-Platt G, Rodriguez-Rodriguez E, et al. Bone changes in alcoholic liver disease. World J Hepatol 2015;7(9):1258–64.

12. Lauing KL, Roper PM, Nauer RK, et al. Acute alcohol exposure impairs fracture healing and deregulates beta-catenin signaling in the fracture callus. Alcohol Clin Exp Res 2012;36(12):2095–103.

13. Lauing KL, Sundaramurthy S, Nauer RK, et al. Exogenous activation of Wnt/beta-catenin signaling attenuates binge alcohol-induced deficient bone fracture healing. Alcohol Alcohol 2014;49(4): 399–408.

14. Obermeyer TS, Yonick D, Lauing K, et al. Mesenchymal stem cells facilitate fracture repair in an alcohol-induced impaired healing model. J Orthop Trauma 2012;26(12):712–8.

15. Roper PM, Abbasnia P, Vuchkovska A, et al. Alcohol-related deficient fracture healing is associated with activation of FoxO transcription factors in mice. J Orthop Res 2016;34(12):2106–15.

16. Stavrou PZ, Ciriello V, Theocharakis S, et al. Prevalence and risk factors for re-interventions following reamed intramedullary tibia nailing. Injury 2016; 47(Suppl 7):S49–52.

17. Torricelli P, Fini M, Giavaresi G, et al. Chronic alcohol abuse and endosseous implants: linkage of in vitro osteoblast dysfunction to titanium osseointegration rate. Toxicology 2008;243(1–2): 138–44.

18. Trevisiol CH, Turner RT, Pfaff JE, et al. Impaired osteoinduction in a rat model for chronic alcohol abuse. Bone 2007;41(2):175–80.

19. Volkmer DL, Sears B, Lauing KL, et al. Antioxidant therapy attenuates deficient bone fracture repair associated with binge alcohol exposure. J Orthop Trauma 2011;25(8):516–21.

20. Giannoudis PV, MacDonald DA, Matthews SJ, et al. Nonunion of the femoral diaphysis. The influence of reaming and non-steroidal anti-inflammatory drugs. J Bone Joint Surg Br 2000;82(5):655–8.

21. Beck A, Krischak G, Sorg T, et al. Influence of diclofenac (group of nonsteroidal anti-inflammatory drugs) on fracture healing. Arch Orthop Trauma Surg 2003;123(7):327–32.

22. Bhattacharyya T, Levin R, Vrahas MS, et al. Nonsteroidal antiinflammatory drugs and nonunion of humeral shaft fractures. Arthritis Rheum 2005;53(3): 364–7.

23. Park SY, Moon SH, Park MS, et al. The effects of ketorolac injected via patient controlled analgesia postoperatively on spinal fusion. Yonsei Med J 2005;46(2):245–51.

24. Daluiski A, Ramsey KE, Shi Y, et al. Cyclooxygenase-2 inhibitors in human skeletal fracture healing. Orthopedics 2006;29(3):259–61.

25. Murnaghan M, Li G, Marsh DR. Nonsteroidal anti-inflammatory drug-induced fracture nonunion: an inhibition of angiogenesis? J Bone Joint Surg Am 2006;88(Suppl 3):140–7.

26. Gerstenfeld LC, Al-Ghawas M, Alkhiary YM, et al. Selective and nonselective cyclooxygenase-2 inhibitors and experimental fracture-healing. Reversibility of effects after short-term treatment. J Bone Joint Surg Am 2007;89(1):114–25.

27. Vuolteenaho K, Moilanen T, Moilanen E. Non-steroidal anti-inflammatory drugs, cyclooxygenase-2 and the bone healing process. Basic Clin Pharmacol Toxicol 2008;102(1):10–4.

28. Boursinos LA, Karachalios T, Poultsides L, et al. Do steroids, conventional non-steroidal anti-inflammatory drugs and selective Cox-2 inhibitors adversely affect fracture healing? J Musculoskelet Neuronal Interact 2009;9(1):44–52.

29. Dodwell ER, Latorre JG, Parisini E, et al. NSAID exposure and risk of nonunion: a meta-analysis of case-control and cohort studies. Calcif Tissue Int 2010;87(3):193–202.

30. Hernandez RK, Do TP, Critchlow CW, et al. Patient-related risk factors for fracture-healing complications in the United Kingdom General Practice Research Database. Acta Orthop 2012;83(6):653–60.

31. Kurmis AP, Kurmis TP, O'Brien JX, et al. The effect of nonsteroidal anti-inflammatory drug administration on acute phase fracture-healing: a review. J Bone Joint Surg Am 2012;94(9):815–23.

32. Pountos I, Georgouli T, Calori GM, et al. Do nonsteroidal anti-inflammatory drugs affect bone healing? A critical analysis. ScientificWorldJournal 2012;2012:606404.

33. Geusens P, Emans PJ, de Jong JJ, et al. NSAIDs and fracture healing. Curr Opin Rheumatol 2013;25(4):524–31.

34. van Esch RW, Kool MM, van As S. NSAIDs can have adverse effects on bone healing. Med Hypotheses 2013;81(2):343–6.

35. Jeffcoach DR, Sams VG, Lawson CM, et al. Nonsteroidal anti-inflammatory drugs' impact on nonunion and infection rates in long-bone fractures. J Trauma Acute Care Surg 2014;76(3):779–83.

36. Giannoudis PV, Hak D, Sanders D, et al. Inflammation, bone healing, and anti-inflammatory drugs: an update. J Orthop Trauma 2015;29(Suppl 12):S6–9.

37. DePeter KC, Blumberg SM, Dienstag Becker S, et al. Does the use of ibuprofen in children with extremity fractures increase their risk for bone healing complications? J Emerg Med 2017;52(4):426–32.

38. Chrastil J, Sampson C, Jones KB, et al. Postoperative opioid administration inhibits bone healing in an animal model. Clin Orthop Relat Res 2013;471(12):4076–81.

39. Chrastil J, Sampson C, Jones KB, et al. Evaluating the affect and reversibility of opioid-induced androgen deficiency in an orthopaedic animal fracture model. Clin Orthop Relat Res 2014;472(6):1964–71.

40. Petrizzi L, Mariscoli M, Valbonetti L, et al. Preliminary study on the effect of parenteral naloxone, alone and in association with calcium gluconate, on bone healing in an ovine "drill hole" model system. BMC Musculoskelet Disord 2007;8:43.

41. Lindenhovius AL, Helmerhorst GT, Schnellen AC, et al. Differences in prescription of narcotic pain medication after operative treatment of hip and ankle fractures in the United States and The Netherlands. J Trauma 2009;67(1):160–4.

42. Kristensson H, Lunden A, Nilsson BE. Fracture incidence and diagnostic roentgen in alcoholics. Acta Orthop Scand 1980;51(2):205–7.

43. Savola O, Niemela O, Hillbom M. Blood alcohol is the best indicator of hazardous alcohol drinking in young adults and working-age patients with trauma. Alcohol Alcohol 2004;39(4):340–5.

44. Sampson HW. Alcohol's harmful effects on bone. Alcohol Health Res World 1998;22(3):190–4.

45. Wezeman FH, Emanuele MA, Emanuele NV, et al. Chronic alcohol consumption during male rat adolescence impairs skeletal development through effects on osteoblast gene expression, bone mineral density, and bone strength. Alcohol Clin Exp Res 1999;23(9):1534–42.

46. Maran A, Zhang M, Spelsberg TC, et al. The dose-response effects of ethanol on the human fetal osteoblastic cell line. J Bone Miner Res 2001;16(2):270–6.

47. Chakkalakal DA, Novak JR, Fritz ED, et al. Inhibition of bone repair in a rat model for chronic and excessive alcohol consumption. Alcohol 2005;36(3):201–14.

48. Clement-Lacroix P, Ai M, Morvan F, et al. Lrp5-independent activation of Wnt signaling by lithium chloride increases bone formation and bone mass in mice. Proc Natl Acad Sci U S A 2005;102(48):17406–11.

49. Day TF, Guo X, Garrett-Beal L, et al. Wnt/beta-catenin signaling in mesenchymal progenitors controls osteoblast and chondrocyte differentiation during vertebrate skeletogenesis. Dev Cell 2005;8(5):739–50.

50. Baksh D, Boland GM, Tuan RS. Cross-talk between Wnt signaling pathways in human mesenchymal stem cells leads to functional antagonism during osteogenic differentiation. J Cell Biochem 2007;101(5):1109–24.

51. Almeida M, Han L, Martin-Millan M, et al. Oxidative stress antagonizes Wnt signaling in osteoblast precursors by diverting beta-catenin from T cell factor-to forkhead box O-mediated transcription. J Biol Chem 2007;282(37):27298–305.

52. Shin SY, Kim CG, Jho EH, et al. Hydrogen peroxide negatively modulates Wnt signaling through down-regulation of beta-catenin. Cancer Lett 2004;212(2): 225–31.

53. Wu D, Cederbaum AI. Alcohol, oxidative stress, and free radical damage. Alcohol Res Health 2003;27(4):277–84.

54. Yost C, Torres M, Miller JR, et al. The axis-inducing activity, stability, and subcellular distribution of beta-catenin is regulated in Xenopus embryos by glycogen synthase kinase 3. Genes Dev 1996; 10(12):1443–54.

55. Weber CE, Kothari AN, Wai PY, et al. Osteopontin mediates an MZF1-TGF-beta1-dependent transformation of mesenchymal stem cells into cancer-associated fibroblasts in breast cancer. Oncogene 2015;34(37):4821–33.

56. Vane JR, Botting RM. Mechanism of action of nonsteroidal anti-inflammatory drugs. Am J Med 1998;104(3a):2S–8S [discussion: 21S–22S].

57. van Ryn J, Pairet M. Clinical experience with cyclooxygenase-2 inhibitors. Inflamm Res 1999;48(5): 247–54.

58. Simon AM, Manigrasso MB, O'Connor JP. Cyclooxygenase 2 function is essential for bone fracture healing. J Bone Miner Res 2002;17(6):963–76.

59. Zhang X, Schwarz EM, Young DA, et al. Cyclooxygenase-2 regulates mesenchymal cell differentiation into the osteoblast lineage and is critically involved in bone repair. J Clin Invest 2002;109(11): 1405–15.

60. Wells G, Shea B, O'Connell D, et al. The Newcastle–Ottawa Scale (NOS) for assessing the quality of nonrandomized studies in meta-analyses. Available at: http://www.ohri.ca/programs/clinical_epidemiology/oxford.htm. Accessed March 12, 2017.

61. Mehallo CJ, Drezner JA, Bytomski JR. Practical management: nonsteroidal antiinflammatory drug (NSAID) use in athletic injuries. Clin J Sport Med 2006;16(2):170–4.

The Importance of Optimizing Acute Pain in the Orthopedic Trauma Patient

CrossMark

Jerry Jones Jr, MD*, Warren Southerland, MD,
Blas Catalani, MD, MPH

KEYWORDS

- Regional anesthesia • Acute pain • Postoperative pain • Orthopedic trauma patient

---

KEY POINTS

- Postoperative pain and opioid consumption can lead to recovery delays and long-term consequences for the surgical patient population.
- Studies have shown that acute pain management is poor, and opioid use as a primary analgesic is not sustainable due to cost, efficacy, and complications.
- Patients with orthopedic trauma are difficult to treat for acute pain, because they are at a greater risk of pain and opioid-related adverse events.
- Optimizing acute pain management in patients with orthopedic trauma is important and can translate into significant positive physiologic and financial outcomes.
- Although multiple examples of outcome improvements are available and are likely viable, outcome success will depend more on systemwide implementation rather than a specific regimen.

BACKGROUND

Over the past 20 years, there has been a dramatic increase in the attention that professional societies and regulatory agencies (American Academy of Orthopaedic Surgeons [AAOS], Eastern Association for the Surgery of Trauma ([EAST], Trauma Anesthesia Society [TAS], World Health Organization [WHO], Agency for Health Care Policy and Research, American Pain Society [APS], American Society of Anesthesiologists [ASA], US Department of Veterans Affairs, Joint Commission on Accreditation of Healthcare Organizations [JCAHCO], International Association for the Study of Pain [IASP], European Pain Federation [EFIC], Australian and New Zealand College of Anesthetists) have given to the importance of the evaluation and treatment of acute pain.[1–12] These groups have affirmed the substantial negative impact of inadequately treated acute pain, and some have specifically acknowledged the "rights" of patients to appropriate pain control (WHO, APS, JCAHCO, IASP).[12] During this same time, the number of reliable acute pain management strategies, techniques, and applications has also grown

---

Disclosure Statement: Dr J. Jones has at present and/or has had within the past 12 months a relevant financial relationship with Infu-Tronix, LLC (consultant), Halyard Health, B Braun USA (consultant, speakers' bureau), Ferrosan Medical Devices Educational Grant: 2017-01-E (consultant, grant/research support, educational grant: 2017-01-E), and U.S. Special Operations Command (USSOCOM) (Cooperative Research and Development Agreement, CRADA: development of Special Operations Peculiar Technologies to bridge USSOCOM capabilities gaps [USSOCOM-SORDAC-ST – 14-01]).

Department of Anesthesiology, The University of Tennessee Health Science Center, 877 Jefferson Avenue, Chandler Building, Suite 600, Memphis, TN 38103, USA
* Corresponding author.
E-mail address: jjones8@uthsc.edu

Orthop Clin N Am 48 (2017) 445–465
http://dx.doi.org/10.1016/j.ocl.2017.06.003
0030-5898/17/© 2017 Elsevier Inc. All rights reserved.

significantly.[13–15] Despite our greater capacity to improve the treatment of acute pain and the increased awareness of the negative financial[16–18] and physiologic[19–25] consequences of inadequately treated acute pain, many patients continue to suffer from moderate, severe, or excruciating acute pain following trauma and surgery.[5,26–32]

In addition, the overreliance on opioids as the primary analgesic agent has become the "status quo" and presents several important barriers to a rapid recovery,[33–35] as well as other important negative long-term consequences.[36] Although opioids may relieve pain in multiple areas of the body simultaneously, often a helpful feature in trauma-related injury, they are not effective analgesics for sources of "dynamic" pain (cough, ambulation) compared with other modalities.[35–37] Further, they do not mitigate central sensitization, a key determinant in the development of chronic pain,[38] and their role in mitigating the negative consequences of the neuroendocrine response[20] is lacking as well. The overreliance on opioids over the past few decades to minimize pain and suffering has led to a prescription opioid epidemic with substantial overdose death and addiction rates, which demonstrate that this strategy is not sustainable (Figs. 1 and 2). Despite this apparent conundrum, there is a growing body of literature that demonstrates significant improvements in patient outcome and health care resource

utilization when acute pain management strategies are improved or optimized by incorporating multimodal analgesia (MMA) strategies.[39–44] Given the growing awareness of significant downstream implications, acute pain management demands greater attention and emphasis in health care.

Patients with orthopedic trauma comprise the full range and extremes of injury severity, age, and health status. It is well known that orthopedic injuries are among the most painful.[26,27] Beyond the common barriers to adequate acute pain treatment previously described in published articles,[45,46] there are additional barriers that may interfere with the provision of optimized acute pain management for patients with orthopedic trauma and deserve special consideration.

Due to the nature of acute traumatic injury itself, the patient demographics of traumatic injury, and the overall management of patients with acute traumatic injury, many patients with orthopedic trauma have a particularly high risk of experiencing short-term and long-term negative consequences related to suboptimally managed acute pain. These consequences are both clinically and financially relevant and result from the undertreatment of acute pain, opioid-related adverse drug events (ORADEs), and prolonged exposure to opioids.[33,34,47–52]

Although there exists a humanitarian interest in relieving the immediate suffering of patients

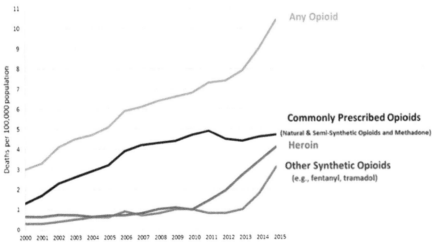

Fig. 1. US trends in opioid-related deaths between 2000 and 2015. Note: commonly prescribed opioids caused a significantly higher rate of deaths over the 15-year period than an illegal substance such as heroin. (*From* Centers for Disease Control and Prevention. National Center for Health Statistics (CDC/NCHS). National Vital Statistics System, Mortality. CDC WONDER, Atlanta, GA: US Department of Health and Human Services, CDC; 2016. Available at: https://wonder.cdc.gov/. Accessed June 15, 2016.)

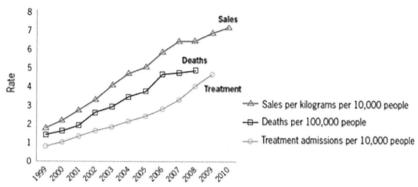

Rates of Prescription Opioid Sales, Death and Substance Abuse Treatment Admissions, 1999–2010

Fig. 2. US trends in the distributions of opioid sales and concomitant deaths/abuse treatment admissions. The need for substance abuse treatment has increased similarly with the increase in sales of prescription opioids. (*Data from* National Vital Statistics System, 1999–2008, Automation of reports and consolidated orders system (ARCOS) of the drug enforcement administration (DEA), 1999–2010; Treatment Episode Data Set, 1999–2009.)

with orthopedic trauma, it has become even more evident that simply increasing pain level monitoring and treating high pain scores with more opioids is not an adequate solution, as this increases the likelihood of numerous harmful effects.[53] This article discusses the scope of the financial and physiologic consequences of inadequately managed acute pain in the patient with orthopedic trauma, reviews examples in the literature of significant outcome differences, and summarizes current guidelines for the management of acute pain. In addition, fundamental institutional elements necessary for replicating positive physiologic and financial outcomes related to optimized acute pain management are highlighted and discussed.

IMPACT OF ACUTE PAIN

Inadequate postoperative pain relief may delay recovery, lead to a prolonged hospital stay, and increase medical costs.[54] The IASP defines pain as "an unpleasant sensory and emotional experience associated with actual or potential tissue damage, or described in terms of such damage."[55] Thus, pain is influenced by not only the discrete nociceptive input that is transmitted centrally but also by cultural expectations and emotional interpretations of the subject. The latter aspect should not be underestimated, as the implications are wide-reaching. Patient surveys consistently indicate that patients fear pain more than they do the possibility that surgery will not alleviate their problems.[3,4] Some patients

delay surgery because of the fear of the associated pain.[4] In fact, the fear of pain may inhibit participation in physical therapy, delay discharge, and affect surgical outcome. Unrelieved acute pain can lead to confusion, especially in patients at risk, resulting in additional testing, monitoring, and increased health care resources.[54]

In the teleologic sense, the recognition of injury through nociceptive input is critically important to the organism.[56] However, the experience of severe pain in humans sets into motion physiologic responses that carry the risk of severe negative acute consequences, as well as long-standing problems, such as the development of chronic pain. The neuroendocrine "stress response" is particularly problematic when the source of severe pain is the scalpel of the surgeon, which is intended to heal and repair a patient. An exaggerated and prolonged neuroendocrine response to acute pain leads to several undesirable consequences, including tachycardia, hypertension, increased work of breathing, intestinal stasis, hypercoagulability, decreased immune surveillance, and a negative nitrogen balance. These conditions may increase the likelihood of acute myocardial infarction, cerebrovascular accident, respiratory failure, ileus, deep venous thrombosis, pulmonary embolism, and confusion.[20] These complications are more likely to occur in patients with certain risk factors or comorbidities, such as advanced age, coronary artery disease, chronic obstructive pulmonary disease, and preexisting dementia.[21,57,58] Morrison and colleagues[59,60] have shown that cognitively intact elderly patients with hip fracture who experienced severe pain were 9 times more likely to suffer from delirium than did patients whose pain was adequately treated. They found that using less than 10 mg of morphine per day resulted in an increased risk (RR = 5.4) of developing delirium. Although opioid-related adverse events and their consequences were not reported in this study, an increased incidence of delirium as well as any of the downstream consequences of delirium (treatment, more tests, increased monitoring, greater length of stay [LOS], delayed recovery, increased incidence of transfer to skilled facilities) will confer a greater financial burden.

Severe pain interferes with pulmonary toilet, ambulation, physical therapy, and occupational therapy. In addition to delaying overall recovery, severe pain leads to immobilization and leaves patients at risk for common postsurgical complications, such as pneumonia,[61] deep vein thrombosis,[62] and catheter-associated urinary tract infection.[63] Severe pain, fear of severe pain,[64] and other circumstances[65] may lead to inhibited joint mobility for extended periods of time. Early mobilization has led to improved outcomes in some patient populations.[66–70] The clinical significance or importance of facilitating early joint mobility and increasing early range of motion through optimized acute pain management and more assertive therapy regimens might be debated because some long-term outcomes produce similar results.[71–73] Dismissing the importance of analgesia-facilitated early joint mobility, however, may predispose some patients to experiencing increased development of adhesive capsulitis,[74] delayed functional rehabilitation,[75–77] or chronic pain conditions.[64] These undesirable outcomes may lengthen hospital stay, necessitate additional procedures and office visits, contribute to long-term morbidity, decrease quality of life, and delay the return to activities of daily living.[64] Severe pain may necessitate significant opioid doses or intubation and mechanical ventilation, both of which can interfere with or preclude serial physical examinations.[75] This is of critical importance in some patients with orthopedic trauma who may be at risk for acute compartment syndrome.[61,78] Severe pain in mechanically ventilated patients may also delay weaning from mechanical ventilation, which additionally interferes with recovery and extends LOS.[20,23,25]

In addition to these immediate physiologic consequences, inadequately managed acute pain may continue pathologically as chronic pain, defined as ongoing acute pain for at least 3 to 6 months' duration.[55] In fact, up to one-third of patients in chronic pain clinics indicate that their chronic pain was the result of trauma or acute pain of surgery.[22,23] The incidence and intensity of chronic pain due to surgery has been well-characterized.[79] There are risk factors specific to individual patients (genetic, psychological, less education, lower socioeconomic status) and types of surgery (amputation, thoracotomy, repeat procedures), which increase the likelihood of pain chronification. One of the most recognized modifiable risk factors for the chronification of acute pain is poorly controlled acute pain.[22,24,38,54,80–84]

Additionally, severe pain is a significant source of patient dissatisfaction. It has been shown that increasing opioid use improves patient satisfaction to a small degree when compared with less use.[53] However, prescribing more opioids to this end can sacrifice patient safety and lead to increased opioid dependence and diversion. Further, beyond increasing physiologic and financial consequences of ORADEs, the patient dissatisfaction related to the ORADEs, which are likely to increase from a more liberal use of opioids, may mitigate some of this potential positive effect of increased opioid use. It has been demonstrated, for example, that if given a choice, patients are willing to sacrifice the quality of analgesia that they receive if this will eliminate the risk of ORADEs. The increasing willingness of patients to trade effective analgesia depends on the ORADE in question. Patients are most willing to sacrifice analgesia to avoid experiencing vomiting, mental cloudiness, itching, and constipation.[85]

The psychological stress and strain brought on by acute pain on the patient and family members involved with a major orthopedic trauma is not insignificant and can result in negative consequences as well. Inadequately controlled acute pain is associated with a high incidence of posttraumatic stress disorder, adjustment disorder, depression, acute stress disorder, and substance abuse.[86] Risk factors for continued opioid use were assessed postoperatively through a questionnaire in adult patients who had orthopedic surgery after suffering a musculoskeletal trauma. Patients with a known history of psychiatric illness, evidence of maladaptive behavior, or history of chronic pain were excluded. Patients with greater signs of posttraumatic psychological stress (those who scored higher for catastrophic thinking, anxiety, posttraumatic stress disorder, and depression) were significantly more likely (P<.001) to report taking opioid pain medications 1 to 2 months after surgery, regardless of injury severity, fracture site, or treating surgeon. Their postsurgical disability severity magnitude was significantly higher (P<.001) than patients not using opioids.[87] Depression and postsurgical pain also can manifest in further complications and increased utilization of health care resources after orthopedic surgery in the long term.[88]

OPIOID UTILIZATION IN ACUTE PAIN AND ITS COMPLICATIONS

The use of opioids for postoperative pain control has been the "status quo" in acute pain management. Patient-controlled analgesia (PCA) use has proven to improve patient satisfaction and decrease pain scores compared with "as needed" opioid administration with an increase in opioid consumption.[89] However, using opioids as a primary analgesic agent often leads to negative physiologic and financial outcomes.[33,34,53,90] The organized efforts to diminish pain and suffering and improve pain scores in one hospital led to a 49% increase in ORADEs and twice the rate of oversedation.[53] The in-hospital odds ratio of cardiopulmonary arrest per 1000 bed-days doubles (odds ratio [OR] 0.92 vs 1.81) when patients are using opioids. The OR nearly doubles again (OR 3.47) when patients also use other sedatives.[91]

The broad effect of opioids is due to their centrally acting mechanism of action. This central effect helps the patient with pain located anywhere in the body but leads to unintended systemic side effects in numerous organ systems. The most critical side effects of opioids are hypotension, oversedation, respiratory depression, and ileus; however, even seemingly minor complications, such as postoperative nausea and vomiting, confusion, constipation, and itching carry with them demonstrable negative consequences. The Joint Commission issued a Sentinel Event Alert in 2012 to warn providers about several identified characteristics that put patients at risk of the respiratory depressant effects of opioids (**Box 1**). Opioids with these groups of patients should be used with even greater caution.[58]

Gastrointestinal complications from opioids are some of the cost common of the ORADEs, and postoperative gastrointestinal dysfunction (PGID) is the most common cause of delayed hospital discharge after surgery of all types. Effective regional anesthetic techniques and other multimodal strategies along with the avoidance of general anesthesia (particularly opioid analgesia) are associated with a reduced incidence of PGID.[80] In a prospective study of patients having bowel surgery, the impact of pain intensity and opioid utilization on incidence of ileus found that total morphine dose (not incision length) was correlated strongly with return of bowel sounds (P = .01), flatus (P = .03), and bowel movement (P = .02).[92] Thus, although minimally invasive surgery has numerous advantages to patients, decreasing opioids may have a more profound effect on PGID. This assertion is corroborated by the findings of Barletta and colleagues[90] that opioid dose is more influential on incidence of ileus than whether surgery is open or laparoscopic. Although the detrimental effect of ileus is twice as common in bowel surgery,[80] many patients with orthopedic trauma are patients with polytrauma who could still be impacted by concomitant injury[93–95] and therefore to the same significant implications of opioid utilization.

The ORADEs far more likely to impact isolated patients with orthopedic trauma are nausea, vomiting, and constipation. The economic consequences of these side effects are discussed elsewhere, but nausea and vomiting are a significant source of patient dissatisfaction and increased LOS.[33,81] Patients with constipation have statistically significant higher hospital admissions, emergency room visits, home health services, nursing home care, physician office visits, other outpatient/ancillary care, and laboratory tests. They also have significantly higher mean all-cause costs for emergency, physician visits, nursing facility, home health, and prescription drug services compared with patients without constipation.[72]

The impact of opioid addiction due to exposure to opioids during episodes of acute pain cannot be overemphasized. In a recent study, 47% (51 of 109) of persons presenting for treatment of oxycodone addiction had their first exposure to opioids through a prescription for pain, and 31% of this subgroup had prior histories of problems with alcohol or another substance.[83]

Although it may be self-evident that exposing patients to high doses of opioids over a long period might increase the likelihood of the development of addiction, even brief exposure to opioids may be enough to lead to addiction. In a retrospective cohort study of opioid-naïve patients having minor surgical procedures, the 27,636 patients (7.1%) who received opioids for less than 7 days (vs no opioid prescription) were 44% more likely to become long-term opioid users within 1 year (OR 1.44; 95%

Box 1
Characteristics of patients who are at higher risk for oversedation and respiratory depression

- Sleep apnea or sleep disorder diagnosis
- Morbid obesity with high risk of sleep apnea
- Snoring
- Older age
  - Risk is 2.8 times higher for age 61 to 70
  - Risk is 5.4 times higher for age 71 to 80
  - Risk is 8.7 times higher for age >80
- No recent opioid use
- After surgery, particularly if upper abdominal or thoracic surgery
- Increased opioid dose requirement or opioid habituation
- Longer length of time receiving general anesthesia during surgery
- Receiving other sedation drugs, such as benzodiazepines, antihistamines, diphenhydramine, sedatives, or other central nervous system depressants
- Preexisting pulmonary or cardiac disease or dysfunction or major organ failure
- Thoracic or other surgical incisions that may impair breathing
- Smoker

Elderly patients and those with significant comorbidities are at increased risk of opioid-related respiratory depression. Note that patients with no opioid exposure as well as those with significant opioid use are both at increased risk as well. It can be particularly difficult to determine safe and effective opioid dosing for patients at either end of this spectrum of opioid use.

© Joint Commission Resources: Safe use of opioids in hospitals. Sentinel Event Alert. 2012;(49):1–5; Oakbrook Terrace, IL: Joint Commission on Accreditation of Healthcare Organizations. Reprinted with permission.

---

confidence interval [CI] 1.39–1.50).[96] Complicating matters further, substance use disorders are significantly more common in patients with orthopedic trauma. Between 40% and 60% of patients sustaining major trauma are affected by substance abuse disorder.[84,97–99] Because the same populations are at high risk for experiencing acute and chronic pain, the prevalence of substance use disorders among persons treated for pain is high, and acute pain management is therefore even more complex and is associated with further risk of addiction.[100]

Beyond the short-term risks and long-term complications of opioid use, opioids are less effective than other available analgesic modalities. In fact, they can increase pain through a paradoxic and poorly understood mechanism referred to as opioid-induced hyperalgesia, which has been associated with very high doses of opioids.[101] Numerous studies have demonstrated that MMA using continuous peripheral nerve blocks (CPNBs)[102] are superior to opioids with regard to effectiveness of analgesia.[103–105] More important than the effectiveness of various analgesic modalities on resting pain scores is the effectiveness with dynamic pain (coughing, deep breathing, getting out of bed, transferring,

ambulating, physical therapy, dressing changes) scores. This metric demonstrates the willingness and ability of the patient to actively participate in recovery, which could mitigate multiple hospital complications[106] related to immobility (pneumonia, deep vein thrombosus), prevent functional decline (muscle strength, nutritional status), and remove barriers to discharge criteria (ambulation distance).[38,107] Tolerating these activities without the need for intravenous (IV) opioids would remove another common barrier to discharge. In a large, prospective single-center analysis of 18,925 consecutive postsurgical patients, D. M. Pöpping and colleagues[35] demonstrated that patient-controlled epidural anesthesia for thoracic and abdominal surgery and CPNB for extremity surgery resulted in significantly lower mean dynamic and resting pain scores (visual analog scale 0–100) compared with PCA (P<.05). Even when studies demonstrate that opioids alone are equivalent to MMA protocols in terms of dynamic pain score, the increased opioid doses necessary to produce this level of analgesia come at the expense of unwanted consequences. In a prospective study comparing PCA to an MMA protocol that did not involve nerve blocks for upper extremity surgery demonstrated equivocal rest and dynamic pain scores during the first 48 hours but found that the patients using PCA experienced more ORADEs on the day of surgery and postoperative day 1 and required significantly more rescue opioids once the PCA was removed. Further, the MMA group reported significantly higher patient satisfaction than the PCA group.[81]

ECONOMIC CONSEQUENCES OF INADEQUATE ACUTE PAIN MANAGEMENT

Calculating the financial impact of various changes to patient care can pose many problems. One is being able to recognize and track all the hard and soft costs that are affected by the change. For example, excessive work duties and deficient nurse staffing leads not only to higher rates of medical errors, it leads to nursing dissatisfaction and turnover.[108] Attending to analgesic needs and complications of opioids is a cumbersome and time-consuming task for nursing staff even with accepted modalities such as an IV PCA[34,109] and reducing nursing interventions because of optimized analgesia practices may permit nursing staff to focus attention on other duties in a timelier fashion and improve job satisfaction. The effect of these changes may not be easily recognized as causal and would be even more difficult to financially quantify. Studies have demonstrated, however, that opioid-sparing techniques reduce nursing time due to reduced need for monitoring and fewer adverse events.[110] The same may occur when the actual cost savings from reducing IV PCAs or IV opioids are not calculated with the cost implications of unrecognized IV PCA costs or from reducing the incidence of ORADEs. Quantifying the marketing and public relations benefits of improved analgesia within a community or recognizing that patients may have chosen the facility primarily due to the lure of optimized analgesia may also go unnoticed.

This issue is complicated further when it is not considered from a global perspective, as financial implications often span numerous departments. That is, some financial implications may appear to be negative when viewed in isolation. For example, the costs due to the increased use of local anesthetic might increase within the pharmacy budget. However, shortening LOS by 2 days or sending patients routinely to a floor bed instead of to an intensive care unit (ICU) or stepdown bed should nullify the concerns. Shortening LOS and facilitating ICU discharge can be achieved simply through MMA

techniques by reducing opioid utilization and their costly negative consequences.[34] Further, by preventing serious complications related to severe pain, for example atelectasis and pneumonia after multiple rib fractures using a continuous paravertebral nerve block or thoracic epidural, patients avoid an extended LOS related to these complications and may decrease the need for additional expenses such as an increased level of monitoring or intubation and ventilation due to severe pulmonary compromise.[111] One study using continuous intercostal nerve blocks in 102 patients with rib fractures reduced LOS from 5.9 days in historical controls to 2.9 days. In patients with hip fracture, another study found decreased LOS and other cost-saving results by implementing an early aggressive pain management protocol using continuous fascia iliaca nerve blocks and facilitating a quicker time to operative repair in patients with hip fracture, which saved approximately $2350 per patient.[40]

Another problem in quantifying economic implications is agreeing on the finite value or even on the validity of individual cost changes to the system. This is particularly true of soft costs. For example, some would debate the financial value of being able to discharge surgery center patients from the post anesthesia care unit (PACU) 1 hour earlier at the end of the day, but not in time to allow for an additional case to be added, as the nurses are still paid until the end of their shift.

Despite the complexities of quantifying some aspects of financial value, any aspect of patient care that can reliably reduce LOS, diminish the need for additional resources, improve patient satisfaction, allow for additional reimbursed charges, or reduce the number and severity of complications to patients will have an enormous positive financial impact for the health care facility. Each of these elements has been shown to be positively affected through the utilization of CPNBs and other multimodal analgesic strategies within organized health care facility programs.

The financial impact of ORADEs is often overlooked, particularly those that are considered "minor" side effects; however, Oderda and colleagues[33] demonstrated that even minor ORADEs remain a significant financial burden to hospitals. In a retrospective review of all surgical patients receiving at least 1 dose of opioids, those patients who experienced an opioid-related adverse drug event (ADE) had median total hospital costs significantly increased by 7.4% (95% CI 3.83–10.96; $P<.001$) and median

LOS increased by 10.3% (95% CI 6.5–14.2; P<.001) compared with matched non-ADE controls. Oderda and colleagues[33] concluded that ORADEs occurred more frequently in patients receiving higher doses of opioids (determined to be only 10 mg of morphine per day) and were associated with an increased risk of experiencing ADEs (OR 1.3; 95% CI 1.07–1.60; P = .01). The top 5 symptoms experienced by patients were nausea/vomiting (49.9%), itching/rash (34.1%), mental status change (16.9%), bradypnea (16.7%), and hypoxia (5.8%). The average cost and LOS increase for orthopedic patients experiencing an ORADE was $861.50 and 0.52 days, respectively.

In a subsequent study selecting for patients experiencing more painful surgical procedures (open and laparoscopic colectomy, laparoscopic cholecystectomy, total abdominal hysterectomy, total hip arthroplasty), Oderda and colleagues[34] discovered even more concerning financial implications when patients experienced ORADEs. In this 2-year, retrospective study of a 450-hospital database of 319,898 patients, 12% of these surgical patients experienced an ORADE and had a higher adjusted mean cost ($22,077 vs $17,370) of $4707 increase (P<.0001) and a greater LOS (7.6 days vs 4.2 days) of 3.4 days (P<.0001). Further, the adjusted OR of being a total cost and LOS outlier were 2.8 and 3.2 times greater in the ORADE group. These patients were also more likely to be readmitted (OR 1.06, 95% CI 1.02–1.09).

Although minor ORADEs carry an unexpected increase in financial burden, patients who suffer from severe complications from ORADEs, such as respiratory distress or oversedation, may require escalation of care, transfer to an ICU, or possibly mechanical ventilation. A meta-analysis of 30,000 patients estimated the incidence of opioid-induced ventilatory impairment for PCA to be 1.2% and for an opioid-containing epidural to be 1.1%.[112,113] Although this is a relatively low complication rate, the number of patients in the United States using a PCA who are harmed by PCA errors is estimated at 6.5%,[114] and the mortality rate resulting from a PCA is estimated to be between 1 in 33,000 and 1 in 338,000.[115]

When patients experience severe pain, and require an IV PCA or when patients experience opioid-induced ventilatory distress, respiratory monitoring needs are often escalated, transfer to stepdown or ICU beds may be required, and LOS may be increased. LOS also will be extended related to ORADEs when increased doses of opioids are used to treat severe

pain.[34] The financial costs involved may be substantial. The average hospital cost in the United States for inpatient stay in a floor bed at a nonprofit hospital is $2025.[116] Transferring to an ICU bed because of concerns of respiratory insufficiency increases costs to $6,667, and the need for mechanical ventilation due to an occurrence of respiratory insufficiency raises the cost to $10,794 for the first day.[117] Subsets of patients who are at increased risk of respiratory depression due to opioid use, such as those identified by the 2012 Joint Commission Sentinel Alert, will require a costlier escalated level of monitoring or will succumb more frequently to costly opioid-induced respiratory complications whenever opioid use is not minimized. Recognizing the costs related to minor and more serious ORADEs, the perception that continuing to use opioids as the primary or sole analgesic is an inexpensive option should be reconsidered (Box 2).

Negative outcomes because of delays in orthopedic procedures[118] or the need for ICU admissions where infection risks are elevated[119] due to nonorthopedic trauma-related injuries are not unexpected with major traumatic injuries. Acute pain management strategies that minimize the need for opioids may have unexpected positive influences on patient care by hastening recovery milestones related to other injuries, obviating the need for a higher level of monitoring, and mitigating delays in subsequent surgical procedures. Consider a patient recovering from an exploratory laparotomy before going on to major orthopedic surgery. Relatively small amounts of opioids after the exploratory laparotomy can lead to complications and delays that could influence the overall hospitalization, LOS, and potentially the outcome of their orthopedic injury. For example, in a retrospective study by Barletta and colleagues,[90] the incidence of ileus and extended LOS was examined in patients after elective colectomy. The odds of developing an ileus were significantly higher when patients received as little as 2 mg or more hydromorphone per day (OR 9.9). This was more relevant than if the surgeon performed the surgery as a laparoscopic procedure (OR 3.1), and the likelihood of ileus increased further with increasing number of days of IV opioids (OR 1.5). They found that the incidence of an increased LOS was associated with development of an ileus (P<.001), 2 mg or more hydromorphone per day (P<.01), and age (P<.005). Asqeirsson and colleagues[120] found that the financial burden of patients who developed an ileus after colectomy surgery increased

---

Box 2
"At-risk" and other patients who may particularly benefit from optimized acute pain management

1. Patients with trauma/surgical procedure or medical condition that historically RESULTS IN MODERATE OR SEVERE PAIN.

2. Patient has an ELEVATED FRAILTY SCORE OR other reasons to be AT INCREASED RISK FOR COMMON POSTOPERATIVE COMPLICATIONS (pneumonia, urinary tract infection, delirium, deep vein thrombosis, acute pulmonary thromboembolism, unplanned intensive care unit admission).

3. Patient is at increased risk of POSTOPERATIVE CONFUSION or postoperative cognitive dysfunction (POCD).

4. Patient is at increased risk for opioid-related adverse drug events (ORADEs), including the following:
   a. RESPIRATORY DEPRESSION/OVERSEDATION
   b. NAUSEA/VOMITING/SLOW RETURN OF BOWEL FUNCTION

5. Patient is at increased risk or potential for OPIOID ABUSE.

6. Patients requiring high doses of OPIOIDS or suffering from severe PAIN that will likely INTERFERE WITH RAPID RECOVERY, discharge home, or return to activities of daily living.

7. Patients requiring high doses of OPIOIDS or suffering from severe PAIN that will likely INTERFERE WITH THE ABILITY TO EXAMINE/MONITOR condition of patient.

8. Patient at increased RISK FOR DEVELOPING CHRONIC PAIN, COMPLEX REGIONAL PAIN SYNDROME, PHANTOM PAIN.

9. DIFFICULT OR COMPLEX ANALGESIA REGIMEN anticipated.

10. OPTIMIZED BLOOD FLOW due to targeted sympathectomy from continuous nerve block.

Early identification of patients at particular risk for opioid-related complications or negative consequences of severe pain is an important step in minimizing adverse physiologic and financial outcomes. This also allows for appropriate allocation of limited hospital resources.

---

costs by $8296 and extended LOS by 4.9 days. These findings show that opioid use, even in small doses, can be directly responsible for significant complications and financial cost. Alternatives to opioid use in the postoperative setting may decrease complications and costs.

Inadequate pain management leads to increased likelihood of emergency room visits and readmission.[41] As payments for care from the Centers for Medicare and Medicaid Services (CMS) are now distributed as a single payment for defined episodes of care (despite additional hospital costs incurred from an unexpected readmission for postoperative pain or from a prolonged LOS due to ORADEs) instead of fee-for-service, hospital savings increase when fewer health care resources are used. Examples of cost reductions through decreased readmission rates was demonstrated by Williams and colleagues[41] with 948 ACL repairs performed over 4 years by using 5 different types of anesthesia with and without the use of single-injection and continuous nerve blocks. When nerve blocks were incorporated into the anesthetic, PACU bypass occurred in 82% of patients (only 2% with general anesthesia alone), and readmission rates dropped enough to cut costs by 12% and save the hospital $98,000 per year. Only 3 patients with nerve blocks were readmitted, and all 3 occurred when the single-shot nerve blocks resolved. Reliably decreased LOS with positive financial consequences was demonstrated through aggressive postoperative pain management and hastening operative fixation in patients with hip fracture. With a focus on opioid reduction and continuous fascia iliaca nerve block infusion initiated early in the emergency department, this coordinated effort saved an average of $2350 per patient after the first year of implementation.[40]

The priority of acute pain management greatly increased for health care facilities since the CMS introduction of the Value-Based Purchasing (VBP) Program in 2010.[121] The Hospital Consumer Assessment of Healthcare Providers and Systems (HCAHPS) survey, a patient questionnaire designed to compare patient perspectives and experience of hospital care, is one of several domains within VBP used to measure hospital performance and reimbursement. Patient satisfaction scores from the random HCAHPS survey now play an enormous part in yearly hospital reimbursement as well as future earnings, and "Satisfaction with Pain Management" is 1 of the 9 rated sections of the HCAHPS survey. In general, hospitals are now graded yearly by CMS based on shifting categories of global quality metrics within the VBP Program. Quality metrics in 2017 include HCAHPS survey (25% of global score in 2017), safety, efficiency and cost reduction, clinical care outcomes, and clinical care processes. Each year, a percentage of CMS payments for services are withheld until the end of the year (3% in 2017) and either paid out or lost depending on VBP model scores. In addition, the amount that hospitals will be paid in the future for individual procedures or admissions are adjusted based on past HCAHPS scores and VBP model results. HCAHPS scores, therefore, have enormous implications, especially for hospitals with a high percentage of Medicare patients.

Although "Satisfaction with Pain Management" is expected to be removed from the overall score calculation by 2018 because of the concern that it could influence the increased prescription of opioids during a national opioid crisis, it will remain publicly reported. This may not diminish the impact of acute pain management on CMS reimbursements as much as one might think at first glance. Patient satisfaction (or experience of care) with several other items that remain on the survey (communication with doctors, communication with nurses, responsiveness of hospital staff, communication about medicines, and communication about discharge information) may still be significantly linked with the effectiveness of acute pain management. For example, when patients experience excellent acute pain management through the utilization of opioid-sparing strategies, CPNBs and MMA, they require fewer nursing interventions to maintain their level of analgesia. Because of this, they experience fewer ORADEs and are more likely to be awake and alert. These 2 circumstances allow nursing staff to attend to other critical responsibilities or to provide more "non–pain-related" interactions with patients, potentially improving the patient-provider relationship. Alert patients are more likely to recall instructions about medications and discharge instructions as well as the time spent with them by surgeons. One large, cross-sectional observational study found that patients rated "Nurse Communication" as the most important of the 9 patient experience measures that correlated most with overall satisfaction.[122]

Alert, comfortable patients are more likely to accelerate their level of activity and to be able to optimize time during physical therapy. This hastens recovery, minimizing the risk of exposure to hospital-acquired infections or common postoperative complications. These aspects of care are elements within other parts of the HCAHPS scores. This scenario may lead to better HCAHPS survey scores related to these additional categories. In fact, one study at a trauma center retrospectively examined HCAHPS responses of 2933 surgical patients and found that postsurgical pain scores were highly correlated with overall patient satisfaction.[123] Studies are needed to verify and quantify these associations.

Further, hospitals may be able report better scores in the "Efficiency and Cost Reduction" category through diminished health care costs per beneficiary by minimizing LOS, decreasing readmissions due to pain, and avoiding costs related to ORADEs. These are all expected outcomes from optimized acute pain management that have been reliably demonstrated in the literature.

ANALGESIC CONSIDERATIONS OF THE PATIENT WITH ORTHOPEDIC TRAUMA

Patients with orthopedic trauma have a multitude of increased risk factors for opioid-related negative consequences and barriers to optimized acute pain management. These reasons can be broken into 3 categories: patient-related, injury-related, and process-related (Table 1). Despite being at comparatively increased risk for experiencing severe acute pain, patients with orthopedic trauma cannot meaningfully benefit from "preemptive analgesia," and may be at an increased risk of developing chronic pain because of an increased exposure to severe pain. Unlike many elective surgeries, most of these patients have already experienced preoperative pain due to the inciting traumatic injury and thereby experienced some degree of peripheral and central sensitization before surgical interventions. This increases the likelihood of intensifying their postoperative pain substantially and in so doing can extend their exposure to opioids. It is this elevation of opioid exposure (frequency and amount) that increases the probability of encountering both minor and serious ORADEs. In addition to the higher rates of opioid use in the United States within the past decade, it is

Table 1
Risk factors and barriers to optimized acute pain management for patients with orthopedic trauma

Patient-Related Factors	Injury-Related Factors	Process-Related Factors
Less likely to be medically optimized	Polytrauma	Antecedent trauma
Greater likelihood of substance use disorder	• *Multiple sources of pain*	• *Central sensitization*
Growing elderly population	• *Delayed analgesia due to ATLS*	• *No "preemptive analgesia"*
Preexisting comorbidities	• *Serial painful examinations*	Medical history incomplete or unknown
Lower socioeconomic and education level	• *Priority given to life threatening conditions*	Unknown opioid and alcohol use
New psychological stressors	Severe pain over extended time period	• *Greater under or overtreatment*
• *Anxiety, PTSD*	• *Greater chronic pain*	Multiple surgical teams
• *> Pain perception*	Monitoring for acute compartment syndrome	• *Greater analgesic gaps*
	• *May limit analgesics*	• *Several staged procedures*
	Postsurgical neurologic examinations	• *Delayed definitive care*
	• *Analgesic gaps*	NPO for bowels, surgery, vent
	Physiologic consequences of trauma	• *Limits PO analgesics*
	• *Limits analgesics*	Multiple dressing changes, drains
	• *Limits analgesic options*	Extended opioid exposure
	Greater tissue swelling, "dirty" wounds	• *Greater tolerance, decreased effectiveness*
	• *More surgeries*	• *Greater ORADEs*
	• *Serial painful procedures*	• *Greater addiction risk*
	• *Delayed definitive care*	• *Greater OIH*
	• *> Risk infection*	Multiple care transitions
	Multiple causes poor sleep	• *Greater analgesic gaps*
	• *Intensifies pain perception*	
	Vent/sedation, TBI	
	• *Limits evaluation/treatment of pain*	

Patients with orthopedic trauma are at increased risk of experiencing severe pain that can be divided into 3 specific causes. At the same time, these patients are often at particular risk for the short-term and long-term negative consequences due to the utilization of opioids.

Abbreviations: ATLS, Advanced Trauma Life Support; NPO, nothing by mouth; OIH, opioid-induced hyperalgesia; ORADE, opioid-related adverse drug event; PO, by mouth; PTSD, posttraumatic stress disorder; TBI, Traumatic Brain Injury.

also recognized that trauma patients have a higher risk of opioid use disorder than the general public,[84,97–99] which complicates opiate utility as an analgesic modality due to drug tolerance.

Surgical intervention in the setting of orthopedic trauma is rarely elective in nature and thus these patients are less likely to be medically optimized at the time of presentation. Provision of expeditious care also can be hindered by language/cultural barriers that limit effective communication. Often, medical care of the trauma patient population is hindered by a variety of factors, including a growing elderly demographic, lower education level of the patients, unknown medical histories, and incomplete medication records that limit the ability to adequately manage the injury in an urgent setting. Additionally, an inability to determine

prior alcohol, opiate, or illicit drug use/abuse/ addiction can result in administration of the medication(s) deemed improper if otherwise informed.[84,97–99] This is particularly relevant in the case of a patient who has tolerance to opioids, or is receiving opiate addiction therapies, resulting in inadequate pain control.

In the trauma care setting, severe pain is often managed with liberal opioid use. Such a strategy is heavily associated with negative outcomes for the patients, such as opioid tolerance and/or addiction.[53] Additionally, the preference for alert mental status to fully evaluate the extent and severity of injury is often difficult to accomplish, as acute pain creates a twofold disadvantage for the provider:

1. It can limit the quality of the medical history obtained and

2. Acute treatment with opiates can sedate the patient and thereby further impair his or her utility as a historian.

Analgesia is often delayed during initial Advanced Trauma Life Support injury evaluation and gaps in analgesia occur due to the priority given to more life-threatening injuries or the need for serial neurologic or other provocative examinations. The early phases of trauma assessment may also limit to the breadth of acute analgesic agents/interventions that may be administered. Examples of such limitations include nonnarcotic medications, such as nonsteroidal anti-inflammatory drugs when concerns for impaired bone healing[124] arise or for acute renal injury in hypovolemic patients; acetaminophen when concerns for acute liver injury or comorbid liver pathologies (eg, cirrhosis) exist; or epidural/neuraxial analgesia if concerns for further hypotension or coagulopathy are present. Still more limitations to effective analgesia arise due to the physiologic consequences of acute trauma, such as hypovolemia, hypotension, inadequate respiratory drive, and changing neurologic status that may worsen with imprudent dosing of narcotic analgesics, especially when sources of active bleeding are not yet fully identified and addressed.

Special consideration must be given to the utility of single-shot and CPNBs in these patients given their efficacy to extend analgesia and to limit the use of opioids. In the setting of high-energy trauma mechanisms, the fear of masking an acute compartment syndrome (ACS) often limits the utilization of this modality. Although the potential risk of masking ACS should be considered, this risk alone should not be the sole determining factor in the decision to implement or avoid perineural analgesia in the setting of orthopedic trauma, especially when the alternative consists of opiate-based therapy that can reliably mask the early symptoms of ACS due to oversedation.[61,78]

Many patients with orthopedic trauma must undergo serialized/staged surgical care involving multiple painful procedures from multiple surgical specialties (eg, plastic surgery, general surgery) and thus are often forced to accept a delay in final resolution of their trauma-related pain. Due to the need for serial dressing changes, repeat debridement and irrigation procedures, or the need to allow for abatement of the associated tissue swelling, definitive surgical interventions are often further delayed in the acute trauma setting. When polytrauma involves the surgical intervention of multiple specialties, it is imperative that a coordinated effort be made to comprehensively address the patient's needs based on clear communication between services to effectively manage patient comfort and pain while not using measures that are counterproductive to the goals of the other specialties involved.

EVIDENCE OF MULTIMODAL ANALGESIA OUTCOMES IN ORTHOPEDIC TRAUMA

MMA has been positively linked to better analgesia,[15,36,41,114,125–132] opioid-sparing,[15,36,125,126,129–136] decreased acuity of postoperative care,[41,132,137] decreased length of hospital stay (faster day surgery and fewer days),[18,41,125,127,131,132,136,137] improved early range of motion,[138–142] improved mobility and recovery,[131,132] decreased persistent pain,[13,143] increased patient satisfaction,[105,128,132,135] and decreased ORADEs.[81,125,132,133,135] In a multitude of clinical scenarios, positive results also have been demonstrated in patients with a multitude of traumatic orthopedic injuries.[13,18,36,81,114,127–133,136,137]

Hip fracture is an area of orthopedic trauma that has been well-studied. Hip fractures are one of the most common orthopedic trauma injuries and are increasing in frequency due to the growing elderly population. Based on studies from the US Agency for Healthcare Research and Quality, 310,000 individuals suffered from hip fractures in 2003.[144] The total number of hip fractures in the world is estimated to be more than 6 million by 2050.[145] In the United States, treatment for hip fractures is projected to cost $10.3 to $15.2 billion per year.[146–153] The 1-year mortality rate for hip fractures varies from 12% to 37%.[114,122,126,127] Based on studies from Chatterton and colleagues,[153] male gender, increasing age, and significant comorbidities are associated with elevated odds of in-hospital mortality, with most deaths caused by respiratory infections (35%), ischemic heart disease (21%), and cardiac failure (13%).

In the emergency room setting, intravenous administration of opioids can provide quick relief for the patient, when compared with intramuscular or oral administrations. However, regional nerve blocks have been proved to be highly effective at minimizing pain without much sedation. Matot and colleagues[159] showed a decrease in preoperative myocardial ischemia events in patients with cardiac disease or high risk for cardiac disease if regional anesthesia (epidural) was implemented instead of conventional analgesia (7 of 34 with conventional analgesia experienced adverse preoperative cardiac events compared with 0 of 34 with regional anesthesia).

Postoperative pain management for patients with hip fracture is crucial to their prognosis. MMA protocols, including regional anesthesia, has shown very promising results in this setting. Using MMA has led to less opioid use, fewer opioid adverse events (thus, fewer ORADEs), a reduction in postoperative pain, improved mobility, and better patient satisfaction.[155–157] The use of postoperative regional anesthesia for patients with hip fracture reduces the incidence of postoperative delirium, when compared with conventional analgesia methods alone.[158] As stated in the AAOS Hip Fracture Guidelines, "neurostimulation, local anesthetics, regional anesthetics, epidural anesthetics, relaxation, combination techniques, and pain protocols have been shown to reduce pain as well as improve satisfaction, improve function, reduce complications, reduce nausea and vomiting, reduce delirium, decrease cardiovascular events, and reduce opiate utilization."[61,157–165] There are a large variety of techniques that result in modest but significant positive improvements in many clinical and patient-centered domains with minimal significant adverse outcomes noted.

AAOS guidelines for acute pain management of hip fractures strongly recommend the use of preoperative regional analgesia, postoperative MMA, immediate intensive physical therapy, use of an interdisciplinary care team for at-risk patients, and optimized nutrition to achieve better patient outcomes.[61,157–165] The significance of these recommendations in the hip fracture population illuminates the importance of effective perioperative analgesia management and should be considered in all patients with orthopedic trauma, given the vast amount of literature already supporting numerous positive outcome metrics from optimized acute pain management in other areas of orthopedic trauma surgery. These AAOS Guidelines for managing patients with hip fracture signify that utilization of opioids as the sole or primary analgesic agent in the acute care of any patient with orthopedic trauma should be relegated to the rare and unusual clinical circumstances precluding multimodal management and regional/neuraxial analgesia techniques. Barring extenuating clinical circumstance, the AAOS Guidelines' emphasis on the importance of balanced analgesia management in hip fractures should be applied to every other patient with orthopedic trauma.

MANAGING ACUTE PAIN WITH CURRENT GUIDELINES

A review of the literature on improving acute pain management reveals a multitude of sometimes conflicting reports of successful practices for patient populations and surgery type. There are multiple discreet practices that have the potential to minimize opioids and improve analgesia in a cost-effective manner.[166] Several societies have recently published new or updated guidelines for managing acute pain with recommendations based on various levels of evidence. There are several generally agreed-on themes that are found in these recent guidelines, which are summarized in **Box 3**.

What is considered adequate or optimal management of acute pain for each health care facility will vary depending on current technical skills, resources, organization, patient population, community standards, and other factors. Whatever starting point and direction that a group plans to go in to optimize acute pain management, the results are more likely to meet with success when there is a focus on the process or program rather than focusing too heavily on a specific technique that is the "best."

What appears clear is that in whatever manner acute pain is managed in a health care facility, there is a cost or value that is associated with that process, and the opportunity to derive tremendous quality and savings is becoming more apparent. More importantly, the ability to determine that value to a health care facility and to compare these financial results across various health care facilities will become much easier with time. The emphasis placed on accountability within the health care system by CMS for quality metrics that are impacted by acute pain management may spread to other private payers in the future.

Overall, there are few in-depth recommendations for specific surgical patient populations,[1,167,168] and these often refer to additional aspects of care that are necessary to improve overall outcome. In fact, most Enhanced Recovery After Surgery (ERAS) protocols indicate that translating individual efforts into meaningful results must do with an entire "system" or combination of processes that are necessary, and the weight of individual variables is not yet determined.[169,170] Measuring compliance with protocols is a key feature to optimizing acute pain and consistently translating these efforts into positive patient outcomes.[166,171]

What appears clear is that the impact of individual techniques that are applied or processes set in place are significantly mitigated if there is not an organized, multidisciplinary approach to implementation with ongoing infrastructure development and interdepartmental

> **Box 3**
> **Acute Pain and Multimodal Analgesia (MMA) guideline summary**
>
> - Use regional analgesia options whenever possible; escalate use based on duration/intensity of pain, and patient conditions:
>   - Incisional Infiltration → Single-Shot Nerve Block → Continuous Peripheral Nerve Block/Epidural
> - Use MMA routinely: do not go straight to intravenous opioids or use as monotherapy
> - Convert to oral opioids as soon as tolerate by mouth
> - SCHEDULE nonopioids UNLESS contraindications
> - SCHEDULE nonopioids EVEN IF little or no pain
> - Use multiple routes for MMA adjuncts
> - Do NOT use multiple routes for opioids
> - Use pharmacologic and nonpharmacologic therapies
> - Consider patient subpopulations at "increased risk"
> - Educate patients/family about analgesia plan and expectations
>
> Routinely modifying your approach to acute pain management by using these criteria will help to minimize the negative consequences of opioids and severe pain. This approach will lead to optimized analgesia and, therefore, greater patient satisfaction, fewer recovery delays, and improved outcomes.

communication.[154,172] Initiation of Acute Pain Services, as recommended by the ASA,[9] have led to improved pain scores and quality of care,[173–175] positive financial outcomes,[175] and better patient satisfaction.[175–181]

SUMMARY

The optimization of acute pain management, especially in the orthopedic trauma population, has significant and far-reaching consequences with regard to improving financial outcomes, patient safety, patient physiologic outcomes, and, importantly, patient satisfaction. Establishing better identification of patients with orthopedic trauma at highest risk for severe acute pain and for higher risk of short-term and long-term consequences due to opioid-related complications and instituting hospital-wide protocols for identified patient subpopulations are important steps in combating these negative and costly consequences. Because of the increases in cost and complications along with the lack of efficacy, the "status quo" of using opioids as the primary analgesic is no longer sustainable. This is certainly true as the transparency in health care continues to increase.

Individual processes and techniques that reliably produce the most effective results in different settings are yet to be fully elucidated, and optimal results are likely to be accomplished by using numerous options. Available and relevant analgesic options in different health care

settings will vary, and multiple options are likely possible to attain superior outcomes. Commitment to hospital-wide screening for "at-risk" patients and improved protocol implementation through an interdisciplinary approach is likely more important than many of the individual aspects of care. As discussed in the guidelines, providing care through an organized acute pain service is optimal when available. APSs are becoming more common across the United States and abroad and continue to demonstrate increased value in various ways, including educating patients and health care facility staff, coordinating care across multiple departments and services, identifying patients at risk for complications due to pain or opioids, and tracking various metrics.

Depending on the approach to acute pain management, the difference in patient outcomes will be substantially different on many fronts, yet many unknowns still exist. Therefore, the management of acute pain will likely continue to demand more and more focus in modern health care and requires an interdisciplinary approach.

REFERENCES

1. American Academy of Orthopaedic Surgeons (AAOS). American Academy of Orthopaedic Surgeons clinical practice guideline on management of hip fractures in the elderly. Rosemont (IL): American Academy of Orthopaedic Surgeons (AAOS); 2014. p. 521.

2. Galvagno SM Jr, Smith CE, Varon AJ, et al. Pain management for blunt thoracic trauma: a joint practice management guideline from the Eastern Association for the Surgery of Trauma and Trauma Anesthesiology Society. J Trauma Acute Care Surg 2016;81(5):936–51.

3. Warfield CA, Kahn CH. Acute pain management: programs in U.S. hospitals and experiences and attitudes among U.S. adults. Anesthesiology 1995;83(5):1090–4.

4. Apfelbaum JL, Chen C, Mehta SS, et al. Postoperative pain experience: results from a national survey suggest postoperative pain continues to be undermanaged. Anesth Analg 2003;97:534–40.

5. Department of Veteran Affairs. Pain management. Washington, DC: Veterans Health Administration (VHA); 2009.

6. Societal Impact of Pain (SIP) platform is under the responsibility of the European Pain Federation (EFIC). Pain as a quality indicator for health care, SIP 2016 policy recommendations. 2016.

7. Chou R, Gordon DB, de Leon-Casasola OA, et al. Management of postoperative pain: a clinical practice guideline from the American Pain Society, the American Society of Regional Anesthesia and Pain Medicine, and the American Society of Anesthesiologists' committee on regional anesthesia, executive committee, and administrative council. J Pain 2016;17(2):131–57.

8. World Health Organization. Scoping Document for WHO Guidelines for the pharmacological treatment of persisting pain in adults with medical illnesses. 2012.

9. American Society of Anesthesiologists Task Force on Acute Pain Management. Practice guidelines for acute pain management in the perioperative setting: an updated report by the American Society of Anesthesiologists Task Force on Acute Pain Management. Anesthesiology 2012;116(2):248–73.

10. Joint Commission on Accreditation of Healthare Organizations. Pain standards for 2001. 2001.

11. Lohman D, Schleifer R, Amon JJ. Access to pain treatment as a human right. BMC Med 2010;8:8.

12. Australian and New Zealand College of Anesthetists. Statement on patients' rights to pain management and associated responsibilities. 2010. PS45.

13. Ong CK, Seymour RA, Lirk P, et al. Combining paracetamol (acetaminophen) with nonsteroidal antiinflammatory drugs: a qualitative systematic review of analgesic efficacy for acute postoperative pain. Anesth Analg 2010;110(4):1170–9.

14. Raza I, Narayanan M, Venkataraju A, et al. Bilateral subpectoral interfascial plane catheters for analgesia for sternal fractures: a case report. Reg Anesth Pain Med 2016;41(5):607–9.

15. Schley M, Topfner S, Wiech K, et al. Continuous brachial plexus blockade in combination with the NMDA receptor antagonist memantine prevents phantom pain in acute traumatic upper limb amputees. Eur J Pain 2007;11(3):299–308.

16. Morrison RS, Magaziner J, McLaughlin MA, et al. The impact of post-operative pain on outcomes following hip fracture. Pain 2003;103(3):303–11.

17. Menendez ME, Ring D. Emergency department visits after hand surgery are common and usually related to pain or wound issues. Clin Orthop Relat Res 2016;474(2):551–6.

18. Hunt KJ, Higgins TF, Carlston CV, et al. Continuous peripheral nerve blockade as postoperative analgesia for open treatment of calcaneal fractures. J Orthop Trauma 2010;24(3):148–55.

19. Young CC, Greenberg MA, Nicassio PM, et al. Transition from acute to chronic pain and disability: a model including cognitive, affective, and trauma factors. J Pain 2008;134(1–2):69–79.

20. Desborough JP. The stress response to trauma and surgery. Br J Anaesth 2000;85(1):109–17.

21. Tetzlaff JE. Cardiovascular consequences of severe acute pain insufficiently-treated severe acute pain has been observed to have multifactorial, deleterious effects—direct and indirect—on the cardiovascular system. Pract pain Manag 2004;4(2):11–3.

22. Eisenach JC. Treatment and preventing chronic pain: a view from the spinal cord. Reg Anesth Pain Med 2006;31(2):146–51.

23. Kehlet H, Jensen TS, Woolf CJ. Persistent postsurgical pain: risk factors and prevention. Lancet 2006;367(9522):1618–25.

24. Joshi GP, Ogunnaike BO. Consequences of inadequate postoperative pain relief and chronic persistent postoperative pain. Anesthesiol Clin North America 2005;23(1):21–36.

25. Moonesinghe SR, Mythen MG, Grocott MP. High-risk surgery: epidemiology & outcomes. Anesth Analg 2011;112(4):891–901.

26. Wu CL, Berenholtz SM, Pronovost PJ, et al. Systematic review and analysis of postdischarge symptoms after outpatient surgery. Anesthesiology 2002;96(4):994–1003.

27. McGrath B, Elgendy H, Chung F, et al. Thirty percent of patients have moderate to severe pain 24 hr after ambulatory surgery: a survey of 5,703 patients. Can J Anaesth 2004;51(9):886–91.

28. Meissner W, Mescha S, Rothaug J, et al. Quality improvement in postoperative pain management: results from the QUIPS project. Dtsch Arztebl Int 2008;105(50):865–70.

29. Dix P, Sandhar B, Murdoch J, et al. Pain on medical wards in a district general hospital. Br J Anaesth 2004;92(2):235–7.

30. Hutchison RW. Challenges in acute post-operative pain management. Am J Health Syst Pharm 2007;64(6 Suppl 4):S2–5.

31. Stanik-Hutt JA, Soeken KL, Belcher AE, et al. Pain experiences of traumatically injured patients in a critical care setting. Am J Crit Care 2001;10:252–9.

32. Sommer M, de Rijke JM, van Kleef M, et al. The prevalence of postoperative pain in a sample of 1490 surgical inpatients. Eur J Anaesthesiol 2008; 25(4):267–74.

33. Oderda GM, Said Q, Evans RS, et al. Opioid-related adverse drug events in surgical hospitalizations: impact on costs and length of stay. Ann Pharmacother 2007;41(3):400–6.

34. Oderda GM, Gan TJ, Johnson BH, et al. Effect of opioid-related adverse events on outcomes in selected surgical patients. J Pain Palliat Care Pharmacother 2013;27(1):62–70.

35. Pöpping DM, Zahn PK, Van Aken HK, et al. Effectiveness and safety of postoperative pain management: a survey of 18 925 consecutive patients between 1998 and 2006 (2nd revision): a database analysis of prospectively raised data. Br J Anaesth 2008;101(6):832–40.

36. Ilfeld BM, Morey TE, Enneking FK. Continuous infraclavicular brachial plexus block for postoperative pain control at home: a randomized, double-blinded, placebo controlled study. Anesthesiology 2002;96(6):1297–304.

37. Kehlet H. Postoperative pain relief—what is the issue? Br J Anaesth 1994;72(4):375–8.

38. Berube M, Choinière M, Laflamme YG, et al. Acute to chronic pain transition in extremity trauma: a narrative review for future preventive interventions (part 1). Int J Orthop Trauma Nurs 2016;23:47–59.

39. Rawal N. Current issues in postoperative pain management. Eur J Anaesthesiol 2016;33(3):160–71.

40. Dulaney-Cripe E, Hadaway S, Bauman R, et al. A continuous infusion fascia iliaca compartment block in hip fracture patients: a pilot study. J Clin Med Res 2012;4(1):45–8.

41. Williams BA, Kentor ML, Vogt MT, et al. Economics of nerve block pain management after anterior cruciate ligament reconstruction: potential hospital cost savings via associated postanesthesia care unit bypass and same-day discharge. Anesthesiology 2004;100(3):697–706.

42. Elia N, Lysakowski C, Tramer MR. Does multimodal analgesia with acetaminophen, nonsteroidal anti-inflammatory drugs, or selective cyclooxygenase-2 inhibitors and patient-controlled analgesia morphine offer advantages over morphine alone? Meta-analysis of randomized trials. Anesthesiology 2005;103(6):1296–304.

43. Horlocker TT, Hebl JR, Kinney MA, et al. Opioid-free analgesia following total knee arthroplasty: A multimodal approach using lumbar plexus block, acetaminophen and ketorolac. Reg Anesth Pain Med 2002;27(1):105–8.

44. White PF, Kehlet H, Neal JM, et al. The role of anesthesiologist in fast-track surgery: from multimodal analgesia to perioperative medical care. Anesth Analg 2007;104(6):1380–96.

45. Drayer RA, Henderson J, Reidenberg M. Barriers to better pain control in hospitalized patients. J Pain Symptom Manage 1999;17(6):434–40.

46. Motov SM, Khan AN. Problems and barriers of pain management in the emergency department: are we ever going to get better? J Pain Res 2008;2:5–11.

47. Latremoliere A, Woolf CJ. Central sensitization: a generator of pain hypersensitivity by central neural plasticity. J Pain 2009;10(9):895–926.

48. Farquhar-Smith WP. Anatomy, physiology and pharmacology of pain. Anaesth Intensive Care Med 2007;9(1):3–7.

49. Kissin I. Preemptive analgesia. Anesthesiology 2000;93(4):1138–43.

50. Hanley MA, Jensen MP, Smith DG, et al. Preamputation pain and acute pain predict chronic pain after lower extremity amputation. J Pain 2007;8(2):102–9.

51. Lawson KM, Back SE, Hartwell KJ, et al. A comparison of trauma profiles among individuals with prescription opioid, nicotine or cocaine dependence. Am J Addict 2013;22(2):127–31.

52. Freeman K, Koewler NJ, Jimenez-Andrade JM, et al. A fracture pain model in the rat: adaptation of a closed femur fracture model to study skeletal pain. Anesthesiology 2008;108(3):473–83.

53. Vila H Jr, Smith RA, Augustyniak MJ, et al. The efficacy and safety of pain management before and after implementation of hospital-wide pain management standards: is patient safety compromised by treatment based solely on numerical pain ratings? Anesth Analg 2005;101(2):474–8.

54. Kehlet H, Holte K. Effect of postoperative analgesia on surgical outcome. Br J Anaesth 2001; 87(1):62–7.

55. Merskey H, Bogduk N. Part III: pain terms, a current list with definitions and notes on usage. In: Merskey H, Lindblom U, Mumford JM, et al, editors. Classification of chronic pain. 2nd edition. Seattle (WA): IASP Press; 1994. p. 209–14.

56. Bonavita V, De Simone R. Pain as an evolutionary necessity. Neurol Sci 2011;32(Suppl 1):S61–6.

57. Makary MA, Segev DL, Pronovost PJ, et al. Frailty as predictor of surgical outcomes in older patients. J Am Coll Surg 2010;210(6):901–8.

58. The Joint Commission. Safe use of opioids in hospitals. Sentinel Event Alert 2012;(49):1–5. Available at: https://www.jointcommission.org/assets/1/18/SEA_49_opioids_8_2_12_final.pdf. Accessed July 13, 2017.

59. Morrison RS, Magaziner J, Gilbert M, et al. Relationship between pain and opioid analgesics on the development of delirium following hip fracture. J Gerontol A Biol Sci Med Sci 2003;58(1):76–81.

60. Warner DO. Preventing postoperative pulmonary complications: the role of the anesthesiologist. Anesthesiology 2000;92:1467–72.

61. Harrington P, Bunola J, Jennings AJ, et al. Acute compartment syndrome masked by intravenous morphine from a patient-controlled analgesia pump. Injury 2000;31:387–9.

62. Toker S, Hak DJ, Morgan SJ. Deep vein thrombosis prophylaxis in trauma patients. Thrombosis 2011;2011:505373.

63. Gould CV, Umscheid CA, Agarwal RK, et al. Healthcare Infection Control Practices Advisory Committee. Infect Control Hosp Epidemiol 2010; 4:319–26.

64. George SZ, Stryker SE. Fear-avoidance beliefs and clinical outcomes for patients seeking outpatient physical therapy for musculoskeletal pain conditions. J Orthop Sports Phys Ther 2011;41(4):249–59.

65. Tanishima T, Yoshimasu N. Development and prevention of frozen shoulder after acute aneurysm surgery. Surg Neurol 1997;48:19–22.

66. Paschos NK, Mitsionis GI, Vasiliadis HS, et al. Comparison of early mobilization protocols in radial head fractures. J Orthop Trauma 2013;27(3):134–9.

67. Beck NA, Ganley TJ, McKay S, et al. T-condylar fractures of the distal humerus in children: does early motion affect final range of motion? J Child Orthop 2014;8:161.

68. Denard PJ, Ladermann A. Immediate versus delayed passive range of motion following total shoulder arthroplasty. J Shoulder Elbow Surg 2016;25(12):1918–24.

69. Parsons BO, Gruson KI, Chen DD, et al. Does slower rehabilitation after arthroscopic rotator cuff repair lead to long-term stiffness? J Shoulder Elbow Surg 2010;19(7):1034–9.

70. Cuff DJ, Pupello DR. Prospective randomized study of arthroscopic rotator cuff repair using an early versus delayed postoperative physical therapy protocol. J Shoulder Elbow Surg 2012; 21(11):1450–5.

71. Kairaluoma PM, Bachmann MS, Rosenberg PH, et al. Preincisional paravertebral block reduces the prevalence of chronic pain after breast surgery. Anesth Analg 2006;103(3):703–8.

72. Dahl JB, Moiniche S. Pre-emptive analgesia. Br Med Bull 2004;71:13–27.

73. Ganapathy S. Continuous nerve blocks for orthopedic injuries. Tech Reg Anesth Pain Manag 2002;6(1):27–32.

74. Kelley MJ, Shaffer MA, Kuhn JE, et al. Shoulder pain and mobility deficits: adhesive capsulitis. J Orthop Sports Phys Ther 2013;43(5):A1–31.

75. Brueilly KE, De Ruyter ML, Ramey KD. Guidelines for physical therapy management of patients with continuous regional analgesia techniques. Acute Care Perspect 2004;13:10–4.

76. Korean Knee Society. Guidelines for the management of postoperative pain after total knee arthroplasty. Knee Surg Relat Res 2012;24(4):201–7.

77. Gadsden J. Regional anesthesia in trauma a case-based approach. Cambridge (United Kingdom): Cambridge University Press; 2012.

78. Azam MQ, Ali MS, Ruwaili MA, et al. Compartment syndrome obscured by post-operative epidural analgesia. Clin Pract 2012;2(1):e19.

79. Perkins FM, Kehlet H. Chronic pain as an outcome of surgery: a review of predictive factors. Anesthesiology 2000;93(4):1123–33.

80. Mythen MG. Postoperative gastrointestinal tract dysfunction. Anesth Analg 2005;100(1):196–204.

81. Lee SK, Lee JW, Choy WS. Is multimodal analgesia as effective as postoperative patient-controlled analgesia following upper extremity surgery? Orthop Traumatol Surg Res 2013;99(8): 895–901.

82. Iyer S, Keith Davis KL, Candrilli S. Opioid use patterns and health care resource utilization in patients prescribed opioid therapy with and without constipation. Manag Care 2010;19(3):44–51.

83. Passik SD, Hays L, Eisner N, et al. Psychiatric and pain characteristics of prescription drug abusers entering drug rehabilitation. J Pain Palliat Care Pharmacother 2006;20(2):5–13.

84. Heinemann Keen M, Donohue R, Schnoll S. Alcohol use by persons with recent spinal cord injury. Arch Phys Med Rehabil 1988;69(8):619–24.

85. Gam TJ, Lubarsky DA, Flood EM, et al. Patient preferences for acute pain treatment. Br J Anaesth 2004;92(5):681–8.

86. Clark ME, Bair MJ, Buckenmaier CC, et al. Pain and combat injuries in soldiers returning from operations Enduring Freedom and Iraqi Freedom: implications for research and practice. J Rehabil Res Dev 2007;44(2):179–94.

87. Helmerhorst GT, Vranceanu AM, Vrahas M, et al. Risk factors for continued opioid use one to two months after surgery for musculoskeletal trauma. J Bone Joint Surg Am 2014;96(6):495–9.

88. Brander V, Gondek S, Martin E, et al. Pain and depression influence outcome 5 years after knee replacement surgery. Clin Orthop Relat Res 2007;464:21–6.

89. McNicol ED, Ferguson MC, Hudcova J. Patient controlled opioid analgesia versus non-patient controlled opioid analgesia for postoperative pain. Cochrane Database Syst Rev 2015;(6):CD003348.

90. Barletta JF, Asgeirsson T, Senagore AJ. Influence of intravenous opioid dose on postoperative ileus. Ann Pharmacother 2011;45(7–8):916–23.

91. Overdyk FJ, Dowling O, Marino J, et al. Association of opioids and sedatives with increased risk of in-hospital cardiopulmonary arrest from an administrative database. PLoS One 2016;11(2):e0150214.

92. Cali RL, Meade PG, Swanson MS, et al. Effect of morphine and incision length on bowel function after colectomy. Dis Colon Rectum 2000;43(2):163–8.

93. Bartkiw MJ, Sethi A, Coniglione F, et al. Civilian gunshot wounds of the hip and pelvis. J Orthop Trauma 2010;24(10):645–52.

94. Eid AM. Non-urogenital abdominal complications associated with fractures of the pelvis. Arch Orthop Trauma Surg 1981;98:35–40.

95. Gao JM, Tian XY, Hu P, et al. Management of severe pelvic fracture associated with injuries of adjacent viscera. Chin J Traumatol 2005;8(1):13–6.

96. Alam A, Gomes T, Zheng H, et al. Long-term analgesic use after low-risk surgery: a retrospective cohort study. Arch Intern Med 2012;172(5):425–30.

97. Norman SB, Tate SR, Anderson KG, et al. Do trauma history and PTSD symptoms influence addiction relapse context? Drug Alcohol Depend 2007;90(1):89–96.

98. Soderstram CA, Smith GS, Dischinger PC. Psychoactive substance use disorders among seriously injured trauma center patients. JAMA 1997;277(22):1769–74.

99. Martins SS, Copersino ML, Soderstrom CA, et al. Sociodemographic characteristics associated with substance use status in a trauma inpatient population. J Addict Dis 2007;26(2):5362.

100. Savage SR, Kirsh KL, Passik SD. Challenges in using opioids to treat pain in persons with substance use disorders. Addict Sci Clin Pract 2008;4(2):4–25.

101. Lee M, Silverman S, Hansen H, et al. A comprehensive review of opioid-induced hyperalgesia. Pain Physician 2011;14(2):145–61.

102. Richman JM, Liu SS, Courpas G, et al. Does continuous peripheral nerve block provide superior pain control to opioids? A meta-analysis. Anesth Analg 2006;102(1):248–57.

103. Ilfeld BM. Continuous peripheral nerve blocks: a review of the published evidence. Anesth Analg 2011;113(4):904–25.

104. Eledjam JJ, Cuvillon P, Capdevila X, et al. Postoperative analgesia by femoral nerve block with ropivacaine 0.2% after major knee surgery: continuous versus patient-controlled techniques. Reg Anesth Pain Med 2002;27(6):604–11.

105. Chelly JE, Gebhard R, Coupe K, et al. Continuous femoral blocks improve recovery and outcome of patients undergoing total knee arthroplasty. J Arthroplasty 2001;16(4):436–45.

106. Ballantyne JC, Carr DB, deFerranti S, et al. The comparative effects of postoperative analgesic therapies on pulmonary outcome: cumulative meta-analyses of randomized, controlled trials. Anesth Analg 1998;86(3):598–612.

107. Fearon KC, Ljungqvist O, Von Meyenfeldt M, et al. Enhanced recovery after surgery: a consensus review of clinical care for patients undergoing colonic surgery. Clin Nutr 2005;24:466–77.

108. Evans C, Schein J, Nelson W, et al. Improving patient and nurse outcomes: a comparison of nurse tasks and time associated with two patient-controlled analgesia modalities using Delphi panels. Pain Manag Nurs 2007;8(2):86–95.

109. Mordin M, Anastassopoulos K, van Breda A, et al. Clinical staff resource use with intravenous patient-controlled analgesia in acute postoperative pain management: results from a multicenter, prospective, observational study. J Perianesth Nurs 2007;22(4):243–55.

110. Philip BK, Reese PR, Burch SP. The economic impact of opioids on postoperative pain management. J Clin Anesth 2002;15(5):354–64.

111. Gadsden J, Warlick A. Regional anesthesia for the trauma patient: improving patient outcomes. Local Reg Anesth 2015;8:45–55.

112. Cashman JN, Dolin SJ. Respiratory and haemodynamic effects of acute postoperative pain management: evidence from published data. Br J Anaesth 2004;93(2):212–23.

113. Hicks RW, Sikirica V, Nelson W, et al. Medication errors involving patient-controlled analgesia. Am J Health Syst Pharm 2008;65(5):429–40.

114. Goldstein RY, Montero N, Jain SK, et al. Efficacy of popliteal block in postoperative pain control after ankle fracture fixation: a prospective randomized study. J Orthop Trauma 2012;26(10):557–61.

115. Vincente KJ, Kada-Bekhaled K, Hillel G, et al. Programming errors contribute to deaths from patient-controlled analgesia: case report and estimate of probability. Can J Anaesth 2003;50(4):328–32.

116. Average cost per inpatient day across 50 states. 2016. Available at: http://www.beckershospital-review.com/lists/average-cost-per-inpatient-day-across-50-states-in-2010.html. Accessed December 2, 2016.

117. Dasta JF, McLaughlin TP, Mody SH, et al. Daily cost of intensive care unit stay: the contribution of mechanical ventilation. Crit Care Med 2005;33(6):1266–71.

118. Lankester BJA, Paterson MP, Capon G, et al. Delays in orthopaedic trauma treatment: setting standards for the time interval between admission and operation. Ann R Coll Surg Engl 2000;82:322–6.

119. Al-Mulhim FA, Baragbah MA, Sadat-Ali M, et al. Prevalence of surgical site infection in orthopedic surgery: a 5-year analysis. Int Surg 2014;99(3):264–8.

120. Asqeirsson T, El-Badawi KI, Mahmood A, et al. Postoperative ileus: it costs more than you expect. J Am Coll Surg 2010;210(2):228–31.

121. Department of Health and Human Services. Centers for Medicare & Medicaid Services. Hospital value-based purchasing. 2016. ICN 907664. Available at: https://www.cms.gov/Outreach-and-Education/Medicare-Learning-Network-MLN/MLNProducts/downloads/Hospital_VBPurchasing_Fact_Sheet_ICN907664.pdf. Accessed January 18, 2017.

122. Elliott MD, Kanouse DE, Edwards CA, et al. Components of care vary in importance for overall patient-reported experience by type of hospitalization. Med Care 2009;47(8):842–9.

123. American Academy of Pain Medicine (AAPM). Postsurgical pain control linked to patient satisfaction with hospital experience. ScienceDaily 2014.

124. Foulke BA, Kendal AR, Murray DW, et al. Fracture healing in the elderly: a review. Maturitas 2016;92:49–55.

125. Hebl JR, Dilger JA, Byer DE, et al. A pre-emptive multimodal pathway featuring peripheral nerve block improves perioperative outcomes after major orthopedic surgery. Reg Anesth Pain Med 2008;33(6):510–7.

126. Derry CJ, Derry S, Moore RA. Single dose oral ibuprofen plus paracetamol (acetaminophen) for acute postoperative pain. Cochrane Database Syst Rev 2013;(6):CD010210.

127. Ilfeld BM, Wright TW, Enneking FK, et al. Total elbow arthroplasty as an outpatient procedure using a continuous infraclavicular nerve block at home: a prospective case report. Reg Anesth Pain Med 2006;31(2):172–6.

128. Elkassabany N, Cai LF, Metha S, et al. Does regional anesthesia improve the quality of postoperative pain management and the quality of recovery in patients undergoing operative repair of tibia and ankle fractures? J Orthop Trauma 2015;29(9):404–9.

129. Ding DY, Manoli A, Galos DK, et al. Continuous popliteal sciatic nerve block versus single injection nerve block for ankle fracture surgery: a prospective randomized comparative trial. J Orthop Trauma 2015;29(9):393–8.

130. Dufeu N, Marchand-Maillet F, Atchabahian A, et al. Efficacy and safety of ultrasound-guided distal blocks for analgesia without motor blockade after ambulatory hand surgery. J Hand Surg Am 2014;39(4):737–43.

131. Sanzone AG. Use of nonopioid analgesics and the impact on patient outcomes. J Orthop Trauma 2016;30:S12–5.

132. Fabi DW. Multimodal analgesia in the hip fracture patients. J Orthop Trauma 2016;30(Suppl 1):S6–11.

133. Mardani-Kivi M, Mobarakeh MK, Kenhani S, et al. Arthroscopic bankart surgery: does gabapentin reduce postoperative pain and opioid consumption? A triple-blinded randomized clinical trial. Orthop Traumatol Surg Res 2016;102(5):549–53.

134. Toms L, McQuay HJ, Derry S, et al. Single dose oral paracetamol (acetaminophen) for postoperative pain in adults. Cochrane Database Syst Rev 2008;(4):CD004602.

135. Singelyn FJ, Ferrant T, Malisse MF, et al. Effects of intravenous patient-controlled analgesia with morphine, continuous epidural analgesia, and continuous femoral nerve sheath block on rehabilitation after unilateral total hip arthroplasty. Reg Anesth Pain Med 2005;30(5):452–7.

136. Cheok CY, Mohamad JA, Ahmad TS. Pain relief for reduction of acute anterior shoulder dislocations: a prospective randomized study comparing intravenous sedation with intra-articular lidocaine. J Orthop Trauma 2011;25(1):5–10.

137. Ilfeld BM, Wright TW, Enneking FK, et al. Joint range of motion after total shoulder arthroplasty with and without a continuous interscalene nerve block: a retrospective, case-control study. Reg Anesth Pain Med 2005;30(5):429–33.

138. Novel protocol with femoral, sciatic nerve blocks for knee stiffness increased range of motion. 2016. Available at: http://www.healio.com/orthopedics/knee/news/print/orthopedics-today/%7Bdd059866-dada-4d14-98e6-e4c0d700f196%7D/novel-protocol-with-femoral-sciatic-nerve-blocks-for-knee-stiffness-increased-range-of-motion. Accessed May 19, 2012.

139. Wanivenhaus F, Tscholl PM, Aguirre JA, et al. Novel protocol for knee mobilization under femoral and sciatic nerve blocks for postoperative knee stiffness. Orthopedics 2016;39(4):e708–14.

140. Ozkan K, Ozcekic AN, Sarar S, et al. Suprascapular nerve block for the treatment of frozen shoulder. Saudi J Anaesth 2012;6(1):52–5.

141. Yilmazlar A, Turker G, Atici T, et al. Functional results of conservative therapy accompanied by interscalene brachial plexus block and patient-controlled analgesia in cases with frozen shoulder. Acta Orthop Traumatol Turc 2010;44(2):105–10.

142. Malhotra N, Madison SJ, Ward SR, et al. Continuous interscalene nerve block following adhesive capsulitis manipulation. Reg Anesth Pain Med 2013;38(2):171–2.

143. Iohom G, Abdalla H, O'Brien J, et al. The associations between severity of early postoperative pain, chronic postsurgical pain and plasma concentration of stable nitric oxide products after breast surgery. Anesth Analg 2006;103(4):995–1000.

144. Agency for Healthcare Research and Quality. Healthcare Cost and Utilization Project. 2017. Available at: www.ahrq.gov/data/hcup. Accessed February 26, 2017.

145. Kannus P, Parkkari J, Sievänen H, et al. Epidemiology of hip fractures. Bone 1996;18(1 Suppl):57S.

146. LaVelle DG. Fractures of hip. In: Canale ST, editor. Campbell's operative orthopaedics. 10th edition. Philadelphia: Mosby; 2003. p. 2873.

147. Huddleston JM, Whitford KJ. Medical care of elderly patients with hip fractures. Mayo Clin Proc 2001;76:295.

148. Cummings SR, Rubin SM, Black D. The future of hip fractures in the United States. Numbers, costs, and potential effects of postmenopausal estrogen. Clin Orthop Relat Res 1990;(252):163.

149. Dy CJ, McCollister KE, Lubarsky DA, et al. An economic evaluation of systems-based strategy to expedite surgical treatment of hip fractures. J Bone Joint Surg Am 2011;93:1326.

150. Wolinsky FD, Fitzgerald JF, Stump TE. The effect of hip fracture on mortality, hospitalization, and functional status: a prospective study. Am J Public Health 1997;87:398.

151. Panula J, Pihlajamaki H, Mattila VM, et al. Mortality and cause of death in hip fracture patients aged 65 or older: a population-based study. BMC Musculoskelet Disord 2011;12:105.

152. LeBlanc ES, Hillier TA, Pedula KL, et al. Hip fracture and increased short-term but not long-term mortality in healthy older women. Arch Intern Med 2011;171:1831.

153. Chatterton BD, Moores TS, Ahmad S, et al. Cause of death and factors associated with early in-hospital mortality after hip fracture. Bone Joint J 2015;97-B(2):246–51.

154. White PF, Kehlet H. Improving postoperative pain management: what are the unresolved issues? Anesthesiology 2010;112(1):220–5.

155. Kang H, Ha YC, Kim JY, et al. Effectiveness of multimodal pain management after bipolar hemiarthroplasty for hip fracture: a randomized, controlled study. J Bone Joint Surg Am 2013;95(4):291–6.

156. Bech RD, Lauritsen J, Ovesen O, et al. Local anaesthetic wound infiltration after internal fixation of femoral neck fractures: a randomized, double-blind clinical trial in 33 patients. Hip Int 2011;21(2):251–9.

157. Tuncer S, Sert OA, Yosunkaya A, et al. Patient-controlled femoral nerve analgesia versus patient controlled intravenous analgesia for postoperative analgesia after trochanteric fracture repair. Acute Pain 2003;4(3–4):105–8.

158. Mouzopoulos G, Vasiliadis G, Lasanianos N, et al. Fascia iliaca block prophylaxis for hip fracture patients at risk for delirium: a randomized placebo-controlled study. J Orthop Traumatol 2009;10(3): 127–33.

159. Matot I, Oppenheim-Eden A, Ratrot R, et al. Preoperative cardiac events in elderly patients with hip fracture randomized to epidural or conventional analgesia. Anesthesiology 2003; 98(1):156–63.

160. Lamb SE, Oldham JA, Morse RE, et al. Neuromuscular stimulation of the quadriceps muscle after hip fracture: a randomized controlled trial. Arch Phys Med Rehabil 2002;83(8):1087–92.

161. Gorodetskyi IG, Gorodnichenko AI, Tursin PS, et al. Non-invasive interactive neurostimulation in the post-operative recovery of patients with a trochanteric fracture of the femur. A randomised, controlled trial. J Bone Joint Surg Br 2007;89(11): 1488–94.

162. Hartmann FV, Novaes MR, de Carvalho MR. Femoral nerve block versus intravenous fentanyl in adult patients with hip fractures–a systematic review. Braz J Anesthesiol 2017;67(1):67–71.

163. Foss NB, Kristensen MT, Kristensen BB, et al. Effect of postoperative epidural analgesia on rehabilitation and pain after hip fracture surgery: a randomized, double-blind, placebo-controlled trial. Anesthesiology 2005;102(6):1197–204.

164. Ogilvie-Harris DJ, Botsford DJ, Hawker RW. Elderly patients with hip fractures: improved outcome with the use of care maps with high-quality medical and nursing protocols. J Orthop Trauma 1993;7(5):428–37.

165. Spansberg NL, Anker-Moller E, Dahl JB, et al. The value of continuous blockade of the lumbar plexus as an adjunct to acetylsalicyclic acid for pain relief after surgery for femoral neck fractures. Eur J Anaesthesiol 1996;13(4):410–2.

166. Nelson G, Kalogera E, Dowdy S. Enhanced recovery pathways in gynecologic oncology. Gynecol Oncol 2014;135:586–94.

167. Neugebauer EA, Wilkinson RC, Kehlet H, et al, PROSPECT Working Group. PROSPECT: a practical method for formulating evidence-based expert recommendations for the management of postoperative pain. Surg Endosc 2007;21:1047–53.

168. Joshi GP, Rawal N, Kehlet H, et al, PROSPECT Collaboration. Evidence-based management of postoperative pain in adults undergoing open inguinal hernia surgery. Br J Surg 2012;99:168–85.

169. Joshi GP, Schug SA, Kehlet H. Procedure-specific pain management and outcome strategies. Best Pract Res Clin Anaesthesiol 2014;28(2):191–201.

170. Kehlet H, Wilmore DW. Multimodal strategies to improve surgical outcome. Am J Surg 2002;183: 630–41.

171. Wijk L, Franzen K, Ljungqvist O, et al. Implementing a structured ERAS Protocol reduces length of stay after abdominal hysterectomy. Acta Obstet Gynecol Scand 2014;93:749–56.

172. Moody AE, Moody CE, Althausen PL. Cost savings opportunities in perioperative management of the patients with orthopaedic trauma MBAP. J Orthop Trauma 2016;30:S7–14.

173. Werner MU, Søholm L, Rotbøll-Nielsen P, et al. Does an acute pain service improve postoperative outcome? Anesth Analg 2002;95(5):1361–72.

174. Paul JE, Buckley N, McLean RF, et al. Hamilton acute pain service safety study: using root cause analysis to reduce the incidence of adverse events. Anesthesiology 2014;120:97–109.

175. Maga J. The safety and financial implications of an acute pain service: in the hospital and beyond. ASA Monitor 2012;76:10–3.

176. Farooq F, Khan R, Ahmed A. Assessment of patient satisfaction with acute pain management service: monitoring quality of care in clinical setting. Indian J Anaesth 2016;60(4):248–52.

177. Katz J, Jackson M, Kavanagh BP, et al. Acute pain after thoracic surgery predicts long-term post-thoracotomy pain. Clin J Pain 1996;12(1):50–5.

178. Godoy Monzon D, Iserson KV, Vazquez JA. Single fascia iliaca compartment block for post-hip fracture pain relief. J Emerg Med 2007;32:257.

179. Abou-Setta AM, Beaupre LA, Rashiq S, et al. Comparative effectiveness of pain management interventions for hip fracture: a systematic review. Ann Intern Med 2011;155:234.

180. Beaudoin FL, Haran JP, Liebmann O. A comparison of ultrasound-guided three-in-one femoral nerve block versus parenteral opioids alone for analgesia in emergency department patients with hip fractures: a randomized controlled trial. Acad Emerg Med 2013;20:584.

181. Ritcey B, Pageau P, Woo MY, et al. Regional nerve blocks for hip and femoral neck fractures in the emergency department: a systematic review. CJEM 2016;18:37.

Pediatrics

Pediatric Perioperative Pain Management

Kaela H. Frizzell, DO[a], Priscilla K. Cavanaugh, MD[b], Martin J. Herman, MD[b],*

KEYWORDS

- Pediatric anesthesia • Pediatric acute pain • Analgesia • Pediatric orthopedic surgery
- Multimodal pain management • Regional anesthesia

KEY POINTS

- Effective pediatric perioperative pain control in patients undergoing orthopedic surgery is crucial for better outcomes, patient comfort, and satisfaction.
- Inadequate management of postoperative pediatric pain may stem from apprehension about serious complications from analgesic medications.
- Initial perioperative pain planning begins with a multidisciplinary meeting between the patient, patient's family, surgeon, and anesthesiologist.
- Acute pain control regimens are customized based on type of surgery, surgical site, age of the patient, anticipated severity of postoperative pain, and patient or family expectations.
- Multimodal strategies and regional anesthesia are useful adjuncts to perioperative analgesia.

INTRODUCTION

Effective perioperative pain management for the pediatric orthopedic patient continues to be challenging. Avoiding the undertreatment of pediatric pain is critical, because inadequate analgesia may lead to longer hospital stays, patient dissatisfaction and an increased risk of morbidity and mortality.[1] Rabbits and colleagues[2] studied children who underwent inpatient surgery and found a significant deterioration in health-related quality of life at 1-month follow-up in children who suffered severe postoperative pain. Yet, evidence suggests that postoperative pediatric pain may not be adequately treated. For optimal outcomes, perioperative pain management should begin with a surgeon-led multidisciplinary discussion with the patient, their parents, and anesthesiologist regarding expectations before surgery.

Perioperative pain management comprises numerous pharmacologic and nonpharmacologic treatment modalities. Treatment modalities include regional and local anesthesia, dissociative anesthesia, and intravenous sedation (deep and conscious). Nonpharmacologic methods include cognitive behavioral interventions and distraction. Acute postoperative pain management regimens are based on the patient, type of orthopedic surgery performed, and current and anticipated postoperative pain. There is a wide diversity of orthopedic surgeries ranging from traumatic fracture care to elective orthopedic surgeries that require different considerations regarding pain management. This article provides an evidence-based overview of preoperative, intraoperative, and postoperative pain management, as well as their possible complications in pediatric orthopedic surgery.

PREOPERATIVE CONSIDERATIONS

Effective pain management begins preoperatively with a thorough assessment of the expectations of both the patient and the patient's family, and the expected level and duration of

---

Conflicts of Interest: The authors declare no conflicts of interest.
[a] Department of Orthopaedic Surgery, Philadelphia College of Osteopathic Medicine, 4170 City Avenue, Philadelphia, PA 19131, USA; [b] Department of Orthopaedic Surgery, Drexel University College of Medicine, St. Christopher's Hospital for Children, 160 East Erie Avenue, Philadelphia, PA 19134, USA
* Corresponding author.
E-mail address: MARTIN1.Herman@tenethealth.com

postoperative pain. The child and parents need to have information regarding the specific surgical procedure, expected severity of pain, and the available nonpharmacological and pharmacologic treatments available provided to them in a clear and simple manner. This discussion ideally takes into account the patient's and family's level of education and is undertaken in their native language.

Premedication

Preoperative premedication reduces patient anxiety, lessens the stress of separation from parents before surgery, and aids in the induction of general anesthesia. Midazolam is the most frequently used drug for pediatric premedication. Midazolam is a short-acting benzodiazepine with a fast onset administered via multiple routes but preferred in its oral form.[3] Oral midazolam (0.5–0.7 mg/kg) provides effective preoperative premedication without a significant risk of respiratory adverse effects.[4] Midazolam is commonly administered 15 to 20 minutes before planned induction. Although midazolam has several beneficial effects, it also has several possible adverse effects, such as excessive sedation, amnesia, restlessness, and cognitive impairment.[5]

Nonpharmacologic Interventions

Nonpharmacologic interventions, which include distractions and relaxation techniques, may help ease the patient's preoperative anxiety regarding the impending surgery and pain. Child life specialists are available at many institutions to provide support through play therapy, music therapy, and other methods. Use of these interventions in the holding area or in the operating room just before induction has been noted to decrease anxiety and improve pain control and patient cooperation.[6] The presence of the parents at induction is another potential strategy but is variably permitted based on institutional preferences. According to Kain and colleagues,[7] children older than 4 years old, those with parents with low anxiety levels, or children with a low baseline level of activity benefit from parental presence during induction.

INTRAOPERATIVE CONSIDERATIONS

Intraoperative pain considerations are an integral aspect of the intraoperative management plan for the pediatric patient. There are numerous opportunities to positively affect the postoperative course: from anesthetic medication options to regional blocks. The ultimate goal is to provide adequate analgesia for treatment, and minimize physical discomfort and negative psychological impact while ensuring the safety and welfare of the child.

General Anesthetics

The new Food and Drug Administration (FDA) warning from December 4, 2016 regarding general anesthetics will certainly cause some parental concerns and questions. The warning states general anesthesia and sedation drugs used in children younger than 3 years of age undergoing anesthesia for more than 3 hours or repeated use of anesthetics "may affect the development of children's brains." The FDA has also issued a labeling change for 11 common general anesthetic and sedative agents that bind to gamma-aminobutyric acid (GABA) or N-methyl-D-aspartate acid (NMDA) receptors, including all anesthetic gases, such as sevoflurane, and intravenous agents, such as propofol, ketamine, barbiturates, and benzodiazepines.[8] Despite this warning, the current literature remains difficult to interpret due to confounding factors. Children who require multiple procedures at this young age often have other sources of anoxic or inflammatory insult to the developing brain that may have caused injury before receiving anesthesia. Recent study has sought to fill the voids in the literature. Davidson and colleagues[9] recently demonstrated that less than an hour of exposure to sevoflurane was not associated with poorer neurodevelopmental outcomes in a randomized controlled trial of infants younger than 60 weeks. Sun and colleagues[10] had similar conclusions in the Pediatric Anesthesia and Neurodevelopment Assessment (PANDA) study, a sibling-matched cohort study of children younger than 36 months. The anesthetic group was exposed to various combinations of inhaled and intravenous anesthetics, including propofol, thiopental, ketamine, and midazolam. There was no difference in IQ scores between siblings when assessed at ages 8 to 15 years. Given this new FDA warning, Andropoulos and Greene[11] recommend an extensive preoperative discussion between parents, surgeons, other physicians, and anesthesiologists about duration of anesthesia, any plans for multiple general anesthetic exposures for multiple procedures, and the risks and benefits of possibly delaying the procedure until after 3 years of age.

Although rare, in the late postoperative period pediatric patients may display maladaptive behavioral changes days, weeks, or even months after surgery. These behaviors include bed wetting, sleep disturbances, temper tantrums, and attention-seeking behavior.[12] A study by Fortier and colleagues[13] found that the presence of preoperative anxiety, sevoflurane-based anesthesia, younger age, emergence delirium, and a lower birth order were found to be risk factors for the development of postoperative maladaptive behavior.

Specific anesthetic agents affecting postoperative pain

Although the anesthesiologist has the ultimate decision regarding choice of anesthetic agents, it is important for the surgeon to be familiar with the medications used, especially in regard to their possible effects on postoperative pain control. General anesthesia is usually administered with various combinations of drugs, including ketamine, propofol, barbiturates, benzodiazepines, opioids, dexmedetomidine, and inhaled agents. A more detailed discussion of the drugs known to have an effect on analgesia perioperatively follows.

Ketamine. Ketamine is a phencyclidine-derived agent that blocks NMDA receptors, providing a dissociative anesthesia that combines sedation, analgesia, and amnesia. It has become a popular means of sedation in the pediatric population and has been shown to be both safe and efficacious in more than 11,000 pediatric subjects.[14] Common side effects include dose-dependent respiratory depression, emergence reactions, nausea, emesis, and clumsiness.[15] Meta-analysis of 35 randomized blinded controlled studies demonstrated use of ketamine intraoperatively decreases pain intensity and analgesic requirement in the postoperative care unit (PACU) but failed to have any further effect on pain intensity and opioid requirement more than 6 hours postoperatively.[16] Prolonged low-dose intravenous infusion of ketamine failed to demonstrate any difference in postoperative opioid use, pain scores, adverse effects of opioids, or length of hospital stay compared with placebo.[17,18]

Alpha-2 agonists. Clonidine acts as an alpha-2 receptor stimulator, likely working on receptors centrally in the spine and locus coerulus. It has been shown to prolong time to first rescue analgesia postoperatively, enhance efficacy of postoperative sedation and analgesia, and reduce propofol requirements for intraoperative sedation. When used in conjunction with bupivacaine intrathecally, clonidine prolongs the duration of both sensory and motor blocks.[19] Transdermal clonidine has also been used in multimodal strategies (see later discussion).

Dexmedetomidine is another alpha-2 receptor agonist that acts centrally on the brainstem by inhibiting release of norepinephrine. It has become a common means of sedation in the intensive care unit but recently has been used as a procedural anesthetic agent as well. Patient's receiving dexmedetomidine require 50% less morphine compared with placebo, and it provides cooperative sedation and easy transition from sleep to waking, important factors in the pediatric patient to minimize psychological trauma from undergoing surgery.[20,21] It is also among the only drugs used for sedation and anesthesia that does not cause neurodegeneration in animal models, which may increase its popularity given the new FDA warning.[11]

Propofol. Propofol is a short-acting intravenous agent commonly used for induction and maintenance of anesthesia in the pediatric population. The drug acts on the GABA receptors, causing central nervous system depression, although its mechanism is not completely understood. Propofol is known to cause pain at the intravenous site during administration, therefore patients are often premedicated with local anesthetic, opioids, or ketamine. Adverse effects also include postoperative nausea and vomiting, and emergence delirium and apnea, although these are less common with propofol use than with inhaled agents. Propofol's effect on analgesia in the pediatric and adult population is still controversial, with many conflicting results; thus further study is warranted.

Inhaled agents. Inhaled agents, such as sevoflurane and desflurane, are also commonly used in the pediatric population for induction and maintenance of anesthesia. They alter activity of neuronal ion channels, including nicotinic acetylcholine, GABA, and glutamate receptors, providing rapid induction and rapid emergence. Malignant hyperthermia, dose-dependent hypotension, nausea vomiting, and apnea are among the inhaled agents' adverse effects.

Emergence agitation or delirium is another dreaded reaction common in the pediatric patient, especially after the use of inhaled agents. It is a rare motor agitation state that can occur shortly after emergence from anesthesia that has been associated with significant preoperative anxiety. During this state, the patient is confused, unaware of his or her surroundings, inconsolable, agitated, kicking, holding their head back, and has an absence of eye contact.[22]

Typically, treatment is supportive unless the patient is at risk for self-injury. If the symptoms are severe, medical intervention may be required with intravenous sedatives, opioids, or propofol. Pharmacologic interventions that have been found to aid in the prevention of emergence delirium include administration of ketamine, propofol (continuously or at the completion of surgery), and intraoperative fentanyl.[23]

Intrathecal Injection

Spinal injections can be performed after induction of general anesthesia before incision or injected directly into the dura during spinal fusion.[24,25] The injection can provide up to 24 hours of pain control following lower extremity surgery.[26] Patients can experience all the adverse effects of intravenous morphine use: nausea, pruritus, urinary retention, and most notably respiratory depression, which can occur up to 24 hours after injection. The hydrophilic nature of morphine and hydromorphone allow them to migrate cephalad and act on the brainstem, increasing risk of dose-dependent adverse reactions.[27] Respiratory monitoring and avoidance of respiratory depressants are recommended. Intrathecal injection with opioids may also reduce blood transfusion requirements, by inducing hypotension during posterior spinal fusion (PSF).[28] In a study of 187 children using low-dose intrathecal morphine (ITM) during a variety of procedures, 81% did not require opioid rescue medications in the first 8 hours postoperatively and 37% had sustained pain relief 24 hours after intrathecal injection.[29] The ideal dosing is unclear but in a study comparing a low dose (5 mcg/kg) with a high dose (15 mcg/kg) and a control group; the low-dose group demonstrated less blood loss, sufficient analgesia, and side effects similar to the control group[30] (Table 1).

Epidural Therapy

Local anesthetics and/or opioids can be injected into the epidural space at a caudal or lumbar level (see Table 1). These are good analgesic options for thoracic, pelvic, and lower extremity surgery. The use of epidural analgesia carries the risk for postoperative nausea, dizziness, hypotension, motor weakness, respiratory depression, and development of an epidural hematoma.[31] Respiratory depression has been demonstrated in 10% to 12% of cases[32,33]; although in a recent study by Ravish and colleagues,[34] lower rates of respiratory depression (7.8%) were seen with lower dose infusions (3–5 mcg/kg of 0.1% ropivacaine ± fentanyl) and

addition of ITM. One of the major side effects with use of local anesthetic is motor blockade, making it inappropriate for use in patients with postoperative concerns for neurologic compromise or compartment syndrome.

Epidural therapy can be given as a single injection or continuous infusion. Continuous infusion can be used for inpatient procedures and remains in place for several days, allowing alteration of volume and concentration of infusion for optimal pain control. A pain consultation service ideally monitors patients frequently for adequacy of pain control and adverse reactions. There are concerns regarding catheter placement and leakage, which can affect efficacy and adverse reactions. Turner and colleagues[35] examined catheter placement in subjects undergoing PSFs by injecting 14 subjects with iohexol contrast in the catheter before obtaining a postoperative chest radiograph. Nine subjects had satisfactory analgesia postoperatively, 7 of which had contrast medium seen in the spinal canal on radiograph. In all 5 subjects (36%) who had inadequate analgesia, there was no contrast visualized within the spinal canal or paravertebral gutter space. Patient-controlled intermittent bolus of epidural infusion is another way to maximize efficacy and minimize adverse reactions. In a recent prospective randomized, double-blind study, there was lower cumulative morphine consumption and less adverse reactions in the patient-controlled group, with no difference in pain scores compared with continuous infusion.[36] The addition of baclofen to epidural infusion has not been proven to provide any analgesic benefit.[37]

Peripheral Nerve Blocks

From 1996 to 2006, the number of orthopedic procedures being performed with a combination of peripheral nerve block and general anesthesia increased from 1.2% to 43%.[38] Ultrasound-guided techniques have expanded their use and allowed for smaller amounts of anesthetic, limiting risk of toxicity.[39] There are several benefits to nerve blocks, including decreased opioid requirements, earlier postoperative return of gastrointestinal function, and attenuation of the stress response caused by surgical procedures.[40] Targeting the innervation of the surgical site allows less use of opioids and avoidance of their systemic effects, making nerve blocks an integral tool for pediatric procedures.

Studies have shown nerve blocks to be safe without lasting neurologic injuries and overall incidence of complications of 0.9 in 1000 regional blocks.[41,42] Most complications

Table 1 Pediatric intrathecal and epidural regimens for spine surgery		
Study	**Route**	**Medication or Dosing**
Erdogan et al,[36] 2016[a]	Epidural	Patient-controlled: morphine 0.2 mg/mL, 0.25 mL/kg morphine bolus and 0.25 mL/kg morphine on demand and no infusion Continuous infusion: morphine 0.2 mg/mL, morphine loading set 0.1 mL/kg, followed by a 0.05 mL/kg/h continuous infusion of morphine, and a 0.025 mL/kg bolus dose of morphine
Sucato et al,[33] 2005	Epidural	Hydromorphone 20 mcg/mL and 0.1% bupivacaine at 0.1–0.2 mL/kg/h
Van Boerum et al,[85] 2000	Epidural	Bupivacaine 0.1% with morphine 0.05 mg/kg/h, additional doses of 0.03 mg/kg/h given by patient-controlled demand
Hong et al,[86] 2017[b]	Epidural or intrathecal	Epidural: bolus with hydromorphone 5 mcg/kg (max 200 mcg) and 1 mcg/kg fentanyl (max 50 mcg), followed by a continuous infusion of 40–60 mcg/h, and patient-controlled bolus doses of 5 mcg Intrathecal: morphine 12 mcg/kg (max 1000 mcg)
Milbrandt et al,[32] 2009[c]	Epidural or intrathecal	Epidural: hydromorphone 10–20 mcg/kg followed by a continuous infusion of hydromorphone 20 mcg/mL bupivacaine 0.1% at an initial rate of 0.1–0.2 mL/kg/h Intrathecal: morphine extended-release 7 mcg/kg and PCA
Ravish et al,[34] 2012[d]	Epidural and intrathecal	Morphine 3–5 mcg/kg followed by ropivacaine 0.1% with or without fentanyl 2 mcg/mL at anesthesia pain service discretion
Cao et al,[19] 2011[e]	Intrathecal	Bupivacaine: 0.5% bupivacaine 0.2–0.4 mg/kg Intrathecal clonidine: 0.5% bupivacaine 0.2–0.4 mg/kg and 1 mcg/kg clonidine IT Intravenous clonidine: 0.5% bupivacaine 0.2–0.4 mg/kg and 1 mcg/kg clonidine IV
Eschertzhuber et al,[30] 2008[f]	Intrathecal	Low dose: morphine 5 mcg/kg and 1 mcg/kg sufentanil High dose: morphine 15 mcg/kg and 1 mcg/kg sufentanil
Gall et al,[24] 2001	Intrathecal	Morphine 2 mcg/kg or Morphine 5 mcg/kg and morphine PCA
Ganesh et al,[29] 2007	Intrathecal	Morphine 4–5 mcg/kg
Goodarzi,[25] 1998	Intrathecal	Morphine 20 mcg/kg and 50 mcg sufentanil

Abbreviations: IV, intravenous; IT, intrathecal; PCA, patient-controlled analgesia.
[a] Equivalent results in both groups with lower morphine consumption in PCA group.
[b] IT morphine group transitioned to oral pain medications sooner with shorter length of stay.
[c] IT provided equal pain relief for first 24 hours with less adverse effects.
[d] Lower pain scores compared with PCA.
[e] IT clonidine prolonged sensory and motor blocks; both IT and IV clonidine reduced postoperative pain.
[f] Equivalent results in low-dose and high-dose groups.

involve failure to place an effective block or inadequate analgesia postoperatively. Serious complications, such as hematoma formation, peripheral nerve injury, and local anesthetic toxicity, are rare.[43] Local anesthetics, however, carry a risk of cardiotoxicity secondary to binding myocardial sodium channels, making appropriate dosing crucial.[44] The precise placement of blocks in children is often done with sedation or after induction of general anesthesia, both of which are proven to be safe techniques.[41]

The smaller caliber of peripheral nerves in children makes them more susceptible to the pharmacologic actions of anesthetic drugs.[45] Blocks can be performed with either a single injection or catheter infusion. Anghelescu and colleagues[46] retrospectively reviewed 179 cases of peripheral nerve block catheters and found only 2 cases of infection, both associated with femoral catheters and catheters in place more than 9 days; therefore, catheter infusion is a good option for procedures with greater expected postoperative pain duration.

Regional considerations

There are numerous regional anesthetic techniques that can be used to help alleviate postoperative pain. It is important for the surgeon to be familiar with the anatomy and pharmacology of the anesthetics to effectively administer the block and/or discuss the appropriate block to be used for a procedure with the anesthesiologist.

Upper extremity

The axillary or brachial plexus block is a safe and effective means of anesthesia and analgesia for procedures below the elbow.[45] The target of the block is the axillary sheath containing the axillary artery and vein, and the radial, median, and ulnar nerves. The musculocutaneous nerve runs outside the sheath and may not be affected by the block, which accounts for the unreliability of this block above the elbow.[15] In addition to the above-mentioned complications, Horner syndrome has been reported, although these complications are rare with axillary blocks.

Lower extremity

The lower extremity may require multiple nerve blocks to anesthetize all areas affected by the procedure. The femoral nerve innervates the dermatomes over the anterior thigh and knee, as well as most of the femur. The knee joint receives innervation from articular branches of the femoral, common peroneal, and saphenous nerves. Femoral nerve blocks are indicated for surgery on the anterior thigh, knee arthroscopy, and anterior cruciate ligament (ACL) reconstruction. The adductor block is growing in popularity because it has less risk of motor block to the adductor and quadriceps muscle, and allows for early mobilization.[47] It is used for procedures on the distal anterior thigh and knee arthroscopy. The saphenous branch of the femoral nerve is anesthetized with this technique. The sciatic nerve block is a good option for knee surgeries as well; especially those involving the posterior thigh, including ACL repairs with hamstring autograft.

Local Anesthesia

The hematoma block is often used in outpatient fracture management and has been shown to be an effective means of perioperative analgesia. Herrera and colleagues[48] retrospectively studied pain control in subjects who received hematoma block with 0.25% bupivacaine after elastic nailing of femoral fractures. The time to first opioid administration was significantly greater in the hematoma group compared with no block. Bulut and colleagues[49] performed a double-blind randomized controlled trial with 20 subjects who received 0.5% bupivacaine via subfascial catheters postoperatively and a control group infused with normal saline. There was a substantial decrease in postoperative pain in the local anesthetic group at 4 to 48 hours. The use of local anesthetic infusion catheters has also been examined in lower extremity surgery for cerebral palsy subjects in a prospective randomized controlled trial. A catheter was tunneled into the incision site and delivered using an infusion device, which provided a steady infusion of anesthetic for 48 hours. Parents reported significantly lower pain scores in the infusion group.[50]

The authors' limited experience with continuous infusion of local anesthetic is that pain control is improved when done in conjunction with opioids; extravasation of the anesthetic may cause skin irritation or chemical burns.

POSTOPERATIVE CONSIDERATIONS

Postoperative pain control has been the focus of recent literature in the pediatric population. Adequate pain control in this population can be difficult due to inadequacies assessing pain, but there are numerous tools that can help make the postoperative experience less traumatic.

Nonopioid Analgesia

Acetaminophen

Acetaminophen is a commonly used medication for pain control in children. It is a weak inhibitor of cyclooxygenase-1 and cyclooxygenase-2 in peripheral tissues, accounting for its lack of anti-inflammatory effect and stronger analgesic and antipyretic properties.[51] Acetaminophen is often preferentially used over ibuprofen in pediatric patients because of the lower risk of side effects, especially Reye syndrome. Acetaminophen's major adverse effects include kidney and/or liver toxicity, especially in patients with prior kidney or liver disease.[52] There has been some concern regarding its link to increased asthma exacerbations but a recent study of 300 children with mild persistent asthma demonstrated no difference in asthma control or incidence of asthma exacerbations compared with ibuprofen.[53] Acetaminophen can be administered orally, rectally or intravenously, and is safe at all ages with weight-based dosing (15 mg/kg/dose) (Table 2). Intravenous acetaminophen has become a popular option for perioperative use. It has been shown to improve early pain scores but has no effect on opioid consumption postoperatively in pediatric and adolescent spine patients.[54]

Table 2
Recommended pediatric dosing for commonly used analgesics

Drug	Dose for Patients <60 kg	Dose for Patients ≥60 kg	Interval	Maximum Dose
Acetaminophen (po)	10–15 mg/kg	650–1000 mg	4–6 h	20–90 mg/kg/d; maximum 3000 mg/d[a]
Ibuprofen (po)	5–10 mg/kg	400–600 mg	6–8 h	40 mg/kg/d
Hydrocodone (po)	0.1–0.15 mg/kg	2.5–10 mg	4–6 h	Caution if combined with acetaminophen
Oxycodone (po)	0.05–0.15 mg/kg	5–10 mg	4–6 h	Caution if combined with acetaminophen
Morphine (po or IV)	po: 0.2–0.5 mg/kg IV: 0.1–0.2 mg/kg	po: 10–30 mg IV: 2–15 mg	po: 4–6 h IV: 2–4 h	Titrate to tolerance
Hydromorphone (po or IV)	po: 0.03–0.08 mg/kg IV: 0.015 mg/kg	po: 1–4 mg IV: 1–2 mg	po: 4–6 h IV: 4–6 h	Titrate to tolerance

Abbreviation: po, by mouth.
[a] Maximum dosing of acetaminophen is controversial; in premature infants 20 mg/kg/d is recommended, Dosing should be based on lean body weight.[56]

Nonsteroidal anti-inflammatory drugs

Nonsteroidal anti-inflammatory drugs (NSAIDs) act as cyclooxygenase inhibitors, decreasing formation of prostaglandins, a major component of the inflammatory response. The earliest age of recommended use varies from 3 to 12 months.[55] NSAIDs have also been shown to be equivalent or superior to acetaminophen for pediatric postoperative pain management.[56] NSAIDs are associated with reversible platelet dysfunction, which may worsen hemostasis or cause bleeding. NSAIDs also carry the risk of upper gastrointestinal bleeding, increasing the risk of an upper gastrointestinal bleed by approximately 2-fold to 4-fold.[57] Despite these adverse effects, ibuprofen is generally safe in the pediatric population. The effect on fracture and wound healing is of particular concern in orthopedic procedures. Intravenous use of ketorolac (0.5 mg/kg/dose) for short-term use (1–3 days) postoperatively is a commonly used modality in many pediatric centers. A study by Kay and colleagues[58] demonstrated no cases of delayed union, malunion, wound, or bleeding complications with use of ketorolac in orthopedic procedures. Ketorolac has been avoided in adult spinal fusion due to concern of postoperative bleeding and pseudoarthrosis, but studies in the pediatric population have shown no difference in pseudoarthrosis compared with placebo and no increased risk of other complications.[59,60]

Gamma-aminobutyric acid analogues

Gabapentin, an oral medication, is structurally similar to the neurotransmitter GABA but its mechanism of analgesia is not fully understood.

It has been used in scoliosis patients undergoing PSF with decreased odds of prolonged intravenous opioid use postoperatively.[61] The need for preoperative dosing and the ideal postoperative regimen of gabapentin in the pediatric population is unclear. A double-blind, randomized controlled trial by Rusy and colleagues[62] demonstrated lower total morphine consumption on the day of surgery through postoperative day 2. In their series, 57 subjects undergoing PSF were given a preoperative dose of gabapentin (15 mg/kg), followed by gabapentin (5 mg/kg/dose) 3 times a day starting the day after surgery for 5 days. Mayell and colleagues[63] examined a single dose of gabapentin 600 mg 1 hour before PSF and found no difference in morphine requirements, pain intensity, or side effects compared with placebo. The investigators postulated the dose may have been too low to be effective for analgesia because the equivalent preoperative dose in the study by Rusy and colleagues[62] would have been gabapentin 825 mg. Gabapentin is an important adjuvant in postoperative pain control, although appropriate dosing and duration of therapy is integral to its efficacy, according to the literature.

Opioid Analgesia

Opioids are effective analgesics that act on receptors in the brain, spinal cord, and peripheral tissues. They are often prescribed postoperatively for pain control and can be administered orally, intravenously, or into the intrathecal and epidural space (see previous discussion). Opioids are associated with several possible adverse effects, including oversedation, urinary retention, pruritus, urticaria, bronchoconstriction, vasodilation, constipation, and postoperative ileus.[64,65] The most commonly prescribed oral opioids in the pediatric population are codeine, hydrocodone, and oxycodone.

Codeine has garnered attention with reports of pediatric deaths after tonsillectomy for obstructive sleep apnea, triggering an FDA warning regarding its use.[66] The liver metabolizes codeine to morphine, with variable rates of metabolism in certain genotypes of the CYPD2D6 subfamily of cytochrome P-450 enzymes.[67] This variability can make codeine ineffective for analgesia in certain patients, and cause life-threatening respiratory depression due to ultrarapid metabolism in others. Therefore, some pediatric hospitals have taken codeine off formulary.

There is a paucity of data in the pediatric population comparing efficacy, adverse effects, and risk of addiction between oral opioids. A double-blind randomized controlled study by Marco and colleagues[68] compared oxycodone (5 mg with acetaminophen) or hydrocodone (5 mg with acetaminophen) use in fracture subjects older than the age of 12 years. The investigators found no difference in pain control and similar adverse effect profiles, although the hydrocodone group experienced higher incidence of constipation. Another double-blind randomized controlled study for musculoskeletal pain also demonstrated no difference in pain control in subjects (aged 21–64 years) who received either oxycodone or acetaminophen (5/325 mg) or hydrocodone or acetaminophen (5/325 mg); adverse reactions occurred more frequently in the oxycodone group.[69] The authors recommend caution with further use of codeine due to the variations of metabolism, but further study is warranted in the pediatric population to determine superiority of other opioids.

Physicians are hesitant to prescribe opioids in the pediatric or adolescent population due to concerns regarding adverse reactions and possible opioid abuse or accidental ingestion. One major concern is the amount to prescribe, especially given the recent notoriety of the opioid crisis, the dramatic increase in opioid addiction, and the subsequent death by overdoses resulting from the use of physician-prescribed opioids. The literature is still unclear about the ideal strategy for opioid use for postoperative pain management in pediatric patients undergoing orthopedic surgery. In a recent prospective study, Grant and colleagues[70] provided some guidance. They identified factors associated with increased narcotic use after PSF: male sex, age (16.4 vs 14 years), higher body-mass index (23.7 vs 19.6 kg/m^2), higher weight, and preoperative pain levels. In their study, subjects were discharged with an average of 61 pills of oxycodone-acetaminophen (5/325 mg). By 4 weeks, postoperative pain scores returned to preoperative levels; therefore, opioid refills at this point were likely not necessary. Interestingly, the number of levels fused, number of osteotomies, self-reported pain tolerance, and surgeon assessment of anticipated narcotic use were not predictive of actual use. The investigators concluded postoperative narcotic dosing could be improved by taking these factors into consideration, although determination of individual narcotic needs remains complex.

Patient-controlled analgesia

Patients experience a variable amount of pain following orthopedic surgery, which is not well predicted by surgeon expectations.[70] Patient-controlled analgesia (PCA) has been shown to be an effective way to treat varying levels of pain in children older than the age of 6 years.[71] In children younger than 6 years or for those that are cognitively impaired, PCA by proxy has been shown to be safe and effective.[72] The benefit of PCA is the ability to maintain opioid levels within a narrower range than intravenous or oral dosing. PCA can be administered with and without basal dosing, which provides even better control of plasma levels of opioid (Table 3). All patients must be closely monitored with use of PCA due to risk of respiratory depression with excessive drug accumulation.

Table 3 Recommendations for dosing of patient-controlled analgesia				
Drug	Dosage	Continuous Infusion[a]	Bolus Dose	Maximum Dose (1 h)
Morphine	1 mg/mL	0.01–0.03 mg	0.01–0.03 mg/kg	0.15 mg/kg
Fentanyl	0.01 mg/mL	0.5–1 mg	0.2–0.3 mcg/kg	4 mcg/kg
Hydromorphone	0.2 mg/mL	3–5 mg	3–5 mcg/kg	20 mcg/kg

Lockout interval for patient-controlled bolus dose usually set for 7 to 12 minutes. Close monitoring for oversedation and respiratory status is recommended while PCA is administered. Dosing should be titrated for effect.
[a] Continuous infusion in addition to the patient-controlled bolus is optional.

Multimodal Pain Strategies

Most studies regarding multimodal pain are in the adult population. Pediatric providers, as a result of the paucity of data in pediatric literature, have been slow to adopt these regimens due to concerns regarding the drug effects in children. Therefore, recent literature has been focused on this topic in efforts to decrease opioid use and its side effects, especially in patients undergoing spinal fusion for scoliosis. Traditional multimodal strategies describe use of acetaminophen, NSAIDs, PCA, and oral opioids. Numerous studies have been directed toward the addition of ketorolac and gabapentin.[73] Administering ketorolac postoperatively decreases the odds of prolonged intravenous opioid use, narcotic-induced gastrointestinal distress, and length of stay after long bone osteotomies, complex foot procedures, and pediatric spinal fusion.[61,74] Transdermal clonidine has also been used in postoperative protocols with lower consumption of PCA morphine.[70,75] Muhly and colleagues[73] recently examined a rapid recovery pathway after spinal fusion for idiopathic scoliosis, using preoperative gabapentin and acetaminophen and postoperative intravenous acetaminophen, hydromorphone PCA, gabapentin, and ketorolac. Despite early transition to oral opioids, discontinuation of PCA, and rapid mobilization, the investigators found daily pain scores remained stable with lower pain scores on the day of and after surgery, as well as decreased length of stay (Table 4). The successes of these multimodal strategies confirm their safety and efficacy.

Table 4
Example of multimodal pain regimen for posterior spinal fusion

Preoperative	• Gabapentin and acetaminophen taken before leaving for hospital
	  ○ Age <12 y and/or <40 kg: gabapentin 15 mg/kg and acetaminophen 12 mg/kg (po)
	  ○ Age ≥12 y and 40–59 kg: gabapentin 600 mg and acetaminophen 650 mg (po)
	  ○ Age ≥12 y and ≥60 kg: gabapentin 900 mg and acetaminophen 1000 mg (po)	

Intraoperative	• Methadone (IV) 0.1–0.2 mg/kg
	• Acetaminophen (IV)
	  ○ Age <12 y and/or <40 kg: 12.5 mg/kg
	  ○ Age ≥12 y and ≥40 kg: 15 mg/kg up to 1000 mg	

Postoperative	• Intravenous analgesia
	  ○ Hydromorphone PCA[a]
	  ○ Hydromorphone (IV q 3 h prn breakthrough pain)[a]
	  ○ Acetaminophen (IV q 6 h for 3 doses)
		• Oral analgesia
		  ○ Gabapentin (po TID)
		    ■ Age <12 y and/or <40 kg: 5 mg/kg
		    ■ Age ≥12 y and 40–59 kg: 200 mg
		    ■ Age ≥12 y and ≥60 kg: 300 mg
		  ○ Diazepam (po q h prn muscle spasm)
		    ■ 0.1 mg/kg (max 5 mg)

POD 1	• Intravenous analgesia
	  ○ Continue hydromorphone PCA, hydromorphone IV prn
	    ■ Stop PCA in afternoon if tolerating po
	  ○ Start ketorolac (IV q 6 h)
	    ■ 0.5 mg/kg (max 30 mg)
	  ○ Discontinue acetaminophen IV after 3rd dose
		• Oral analgesia
		  ○ Continue gabapentin, diazepam prn
		  ○ Start acetaminophen (po q 4 h prn)
		  ○ Start oxycodone (po q 4 h prn)[a]
		    ■ When tolerating diet

POD 2	• Intravenous analgesia
	  ○ Continue hydromorphone IV prn and ketorolac (max 8 doses)
	  ○ Discontinue PCA
		• Oral analgesia
		  ○ Continue gabapentin, diazepam prn, acetaminophen prn, oxycodone prn

POD 3 or day of discharge	• Intravenous analgesia
	  ○ Continue hydromorphone IV prn
	  ○ Discontinue ketorolac after 8th dose
		• Oral analgesia
		  ○ Continue gabapentin, diazepam prn, acetaminophen prn, oxycodone prn

Example of a multimodal pain regimen used for PSF by Muhly et al. in their rapid recovery pathway, resulting in earlier mobilization and shorter length of stay without an increase in pain scores or readmissions.

Abbreviations: POD, postoperative day; prn, as needed; q, every; TID, 3 times a day.

[a] All opioid dosing was conducted by a pain service.

Data from Muhly WT, Sankar WN, Ryan K, et al. Rapid recovery pathway after spinal fusion for idiopathic scoliosis. Pediatrics 2016;137(4):[pii:e20151568].

Psychological Interventions or Factors

Although not the primary intervention in postoperative pain control, it is important to consider psychological factors and possible interventions. Studies in adolescents and adults have demonstrated association between anxiety and depression and difficulty with postoperative pain control.[76,77] Patient-perceived control of their situation has also been shown to affect pain perception and medication use.[78] In a meta-analysis of perioperative psychological interventions, Davidson and colleagues[79] found interventions such as watching movies, video games, and listening to music were effective at reduction of pain in the immediate postoperative period (less than 24 hours). Given the benign nature of these interventions, it could be useful to suggest them as an adjunct to other pain control methods.

SPECIAL CONSIDERATIONS
Pain Control After Surgery for High Risk Fractures

High-energy injury and specific fracture patterns (ie, supracondylar humerus fractures and tibial shaft fractures) have a higher risk of compartment syndrome. In children, anxiety, agitation, and increased need for analgesia are the most sensitive findings of impending compartment syndrome. In these patients it is paramount to be able to identify an impending compartment syndrome, therefore oversedation with opioids is of great concern. A study by Swanson and colleagues[80] retrospectively evaluated 217 subjects who underwent closed reduction and percutaneous pinning for supracondylar humerus fracture who received either acetaminophen or opioids for analgesia postoperatively. They found no significant difference in pain scores and that demonstrated that acetaminophen is an effective means of pain control after this surgery, avoiding the risk of oversedation (**Fig. 1**). Intra-articular elbow injection was described by Georgopoulos and colleagues[81] in a randomized controlled trial after percutaneous pinning for supracondylar humerus fracture. Compared with the control group, subjects who received 0.25% bupivacaine (4–5 mL) intra-articular injection after fracture fixation had improved pain control postoperatively and no significant difference in complications. The use of regional anesthesia in these fractures has also been described with decreased intraoperative opioid consumption and PACU pain scores with no cases of compartment syndrome.[82] Historically, there has been debate regarding the use of regional anesthesia when there is concern for compartment syndrome, although recent case reports

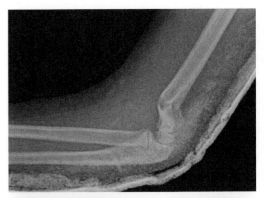

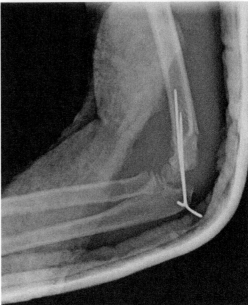

Fig. 1. Radiographs of a supracondylar humerus fracture with a high risk for compartment syndrome before (*upper*) and after (*lower*) closed reduction and percutaneous pinning. Swanson and colleagues examined the use of acetaminophen alone for pain control after closed reduction and percutaneous pinning for supracondylar humerus fractures. After a retrospective review of 217 subjects, the investigators concluded acetaminophen alone was just as effective as narcotic analgesics without the risk of oversedation. (*Data from* Swanson CE, Chang K, Schleyer E, et al. Postoperative pain control after supracondylar humerus fracture fixation. J Pediatr Orthop 2012;32(5):452–5.)

have postulated ischemic pain is not masked by the nerve blocks.[83] Given the multitude of safer options with adequate analgesia, the authors generally do not use regional anesthesia in this patient population.

FUTURE DIRECTIONS

Many pediatric centers are implementing pain services to help insure adequate pain control in the pediatric population. In the pediatric spine surgery literature, pain services are a means to better coordinated multimodal regimens and, more recently, as a means of identifying patients who may be undermedicated.[34,73,84] Further implementation of these pain services can assist surgeons in managing perioperative pain and better identify regimens that improve patient comfort and outcomes.[73] In conjunction with this team approach, it is imperative to begin discussions of opioid use and proper disposal with parents and patients to help prevent abuse in this vulnerable patient population.[70]

SUMMARY

There are numerous safe and efficacious options for the perioperative management of pain in the pediatric population. It is paramount to understand the appropriate uses and safety profile of all the modalities used. Although opioids are safe in the pediatric population, multimodal strategies, as well as regional analgesics, provide opportunities to decrease the need for opioid use and thus the associated adverse reactions.

REFERENCES

1. Haeller G, Laroche T, Clergue F. Morbidity in anaesthesia: today and tomorrow. Best Prac Res Clin Anaesthesiol 2011;25(2):123–32.
2. Rabbits JA, Palermo TM, Zhou C, et al. Pain and health-related quality of life after pediatric inpatient surgery. J Pain 2015;12:1334–41.
3. Kain ZN, Hofstadter MB, Mayes LC, et al. Midazolam: effects on amnesia and anxiety in children. Anesthesiology 2000;93:676–84.
4. Feld LH, Negus JB, White PF. Oral midazolam preanesthetic medication in pediatric outpatients. Anesthesiology 1990;73:831–4.
5. Acil M, Basgul E, Celiker V, et al. Perioperative effects of melatonin and midazolam premedication on sedation, orientation, anxiety scores and psychomotor performance. Eur J Anaesthesiol 2004; 21:553–7.
6. Brewer S, Gleditsch SL, Syblik D, et al. Pediatric anxiety: child life intervention in day surgery. J Pediatr Nurs 2006;21(1):13–22.
7. Kain ZN, Mayes LC, Caramico LA, et al. Parental presence during induction of anesthesia. A randomized controlled trial. Anesthesiology 1996; 84(5):1060–7.
8. U.S. Food and Drug Administration. FDA Drug Safety Communication: FDA review results in new warnings about using general anesthetics and sedation drugs in young children and pregnant women. In: Drug Safety and Availability. 2016. Available at: https://www.fda.gov/Drugs/DrugSafety/ucm532356.htm. Acesssed March 17, 2017.
9. Davidson AJ, Disma N, de Graaff JC, et al. Neurodevelopmental outcome at 2 years of age after general anaesthesia and awake-regional anaesthesia in infancy (GAS): an international multicentre, randomised controlled trial. Lancet 2016; 387(10015):239–50.
10. Sun LS, Li G, Miller TL, et al. Association between a single general anesthesia exposure before age 36 months and neurocognitive outcomes in later childhood. JAMA 2016;315(21):2312–20.
11. Andropoulos DB, Greene MF. Anesthesia and developing brains - implications of the FDA warning. N Engl J Med 2017;376(10):905–7.
12. Sadhasivam S, Cohen LL, Hosu L, et al. Real-time assessment of perioperative behaviors in children and parents: development and validation of the perioperative adult child behavioral interaction scale. Anesth Analg 2010;110:1109–15.
13. Fortier MA, Del Rosario AM, Rosenbaum A, et al. Beyond pain: predictors of postoperative maladaptive behavior change in children. Paediatr Anaesth 2010;20:445–53. Top of Form.
14. Green SM, Johnson NE. Ketamine sedation for pediatric procedures: part 2, review and implications. Ann Emerg Med 1990;19(9):1033–46.
15. McCarty EC, Mencio GA, Green NE. Anesthesia and analgesia for the ambulatory management of fractures in children. J Am Acad Orthop Surg 1999;7(2):81–91.
16. Dahmani S, Michelet D, Abback PS, et al. Ketamine for perioperative pain management in children: a meta-analysis of published studies. Paediatr Anaesth 2011;21(6):636–52.
17. Pestieau SR, Finkel JC, Junqueira MM, et al. Prolonged perioperative infusion of low-dose ketamine does not alter opioid use after pediatric scoliosis surgery. Paediatr Anaesth 2014;24(6): 582–90.
18. Perelló M, Artés D, Pascuets C, et al. Prolonged perioperative low-dose ketamine does not improve short and long-term outcomes after pediatric idiopathic scoliosis surgery. Spine (Phila Pa 1976) 2017; 42(5):E304–12.
19. Cao JP, Miao XY, Liu J, et al. An evaluation of intrathecal bupivacaine combined with intrathecal or intravenous clonidine in children undergoing orthopedic surgery: a randomized double-blinded study. Paediatr Anaesth 2011;21(4):399–405.
20. Bhana N, Goa KL, McClellan KJ. Dexmedetomidine. Drugs 2000;59(2):263–8 [discussion: 269–70].
21. Martin E, Ramsay G, Mantz J, et al. The role of the alpha2-adrenoceptor agonist dexmedetomidine in postsurgical sedation in the intensive care unit. J Intensive Care Med 2003;18(1):29.

22. Voepel-Lewis T, Malviya S, Tait AR. A prospective cohort study of emergence agitation in the pediatric postanesthesia care unit. Anesth Analg 2003;96:1625–30.

23. Dahmani S, Stany I, Brasher C, et al. Pharmacological prevention of sevoflurane and desflurane-related emergence agitation in children: a meta-analysis of published studies. Br J Anaesth 2010;104:216–23.

24. Gall O, Aubineau JV, Bernière J, et al. Analgesic effect of low-dose intrathecal morphine after spinal fusion in children. Anesthesiology 2001;94(3):447–52.

25. Goodarzi M. The advantages of intrathecal opioids for spinal fusion in children. Paediatr Anaesth 1998;8(2):131–4.

26. Coté CJ, Lerman J, Todres ID. A practice of anesthesia for infants and children. 4th edition. Philadelphia: Saunders/Elsevier; 2009.

27. Rathmell JP, Lair TR, Nauman B. The role of intrathecal drugs in the treatment of acute pain. Anesth Analg 2005;101(5 Suppl):S30–43.

28. Lesniak AB, Tremblay P, Dalens BJ, et al. Intrathecal morphine reduces blood loss during idiopathic scoliosis surgery: retrospective study of 256 pediatric cases. Paediatr Anaesth 2013;23(3):265–70.

29. Ganesh A, Kim A, Casale P, et al. Low-dose intrathecal morphine for postoperative analgesia in children. Anesth Analg 2007;104(2):271–6.

30. Eschertzhuber S, Hohlrieder M, Keller C, et al. Comparison of high- and low-dose intrathecal morphine for spinal fusion in children. Br J Anaesth 2008;100(4):538–43.

31. Viscusi ER. Emerging techniques in the management of acute pain: epidural analgesia. Anesth Analg 2005;101(5 Suppl):S23–9.

32. Milbrandt TA, Singhal M, Minter C, et al. A comparison of three methods of pain control for posterior spinal fusions in adolescent idiopathic scoliosis. Spine (Phila Pa 1976) 2009;34(14):1499–503.

33. Sucato DJ, Duey-Holtz A, Elerson E, et al. Postoperative analgesia following surgical correction for adolescent idiopathic scoliosis: a comparison of continuous epidural analgesia and patient-controlled analgesia. Spine (Phila Pa 1976) 2005;30(2):211–7.

34. Ravish M, Muldowney B, Becker A, et al. Pain management in patients with adolescent idiopathic scoliosis undergoing posterior spinal fusion: combined intrathecal morphine and continuous epidural versus PCA. J Pediatr Orthop 2012;32(8):799–804.

35. Turner A, Lee J, Mitchell R, et al. The efficacy of surgically placed epidural catheters for analgesia after posterior spinal surgery. Anaesthesia 2000;55(4):370–3.

36. Erdogan MA, Ozgul U, Uçar M, et al. Patient-controlled intermittent epidural bolus versus epidural infusion for posterior spinal fusion after adolescent idiopathic scoliosis: prospective randomized double-blinded Study. Spine (Phila Pa 1976) 2016;42:882–6.

37. Nemeth BA, Montero RJ, Halanski MA, et al. Epidural baclofen for the management of postoperative pain in children with cerebral palsy. J Pediatr Orthop 2015;35(6):571–5.

38. Kuo C, Edwards A, Mazumdar M, et al. Regional anesthesia for children undergoing orthopedic ambulatory surgeries in the United States, 1996-2006. HSS J 2012;8(2):133–6.

39. Tsui BC, Pillay JJ. Evidence-based medicine: assessment of ultrasound imaging for regional anesthesia in infants, children, and adolescents. Reg Anesth Pain Med 2010;35(2 Suppl):S47–54.

40. Rubin K, Sullivan D, Sadhasivam S. Are peripheral and neuraxial blocks with ultrasound guidance more effective and safe in children? Paediatr Anaesth 2009;19(2):92–6.

41. Giaufré E, Dalens B, Gombert A. Epidemiology and morbidity of regional anesthesia in children: a one-year prospective survey of the French-Language Society of Pediatric Anesthesiologists. Anesth Analg 1996;83(5):904–12.

42. DeVera HV, Furukawa KT, Matson MD, et al. Regional techniques as an adjunct to general anesthesia for pediatric extremity and spine surgery. J Pediatr Orthop 2006;26(6):801–4.

43. Dalens BJ. Regional anesthesia in infants, children, and adolescents. London: Williams & Wilkins; 1995.

44. Rodriguez E, Jordan R. Contemporary trends in pediatric sedation and analgesia. Emerg Med Clin North Am 2002;20:199–222.

45. Wedel DJ, Krohn JS, Hall JA. Brachial plexus anesthesia in pediatric patients. Mayo Clin Proc 1991;66(6):583–8.

46. Anghelescu DL, Harris BL, Faughnan LG, et al. Risk of catheter-associated infection in young hematology/oncology patients receiving long-term peripheral nerve blocks. Paediatr Anaesth 2012;22(11):1110–6.

47. Muhly WT, Gurnaney HG, Ganesh A. Regional anesthesia for pediatric knee surgery: a review of the indications, procedures, outcomes, safety, and challenges. Local Reg Anesth 2015;8:85–91.

48. Herrera JA, Wall EJ, Foad SL. Hematoma block reduces narcotic pain medication after femoral elastic nailing in children. J Pediatr Orthop 2004;24(3):254–6.

49. Bulut T, Yilmazlar A, Yavascaoglu B, et al. The effect of local anaesthetic on post-operative pain with wound instillation via a catheter for paediatric orthopaedic extremity surgery. J Child Orthop 2011;5(3):179–85.

50. Muthusamy K, Recktenwall SM, Friesen RM, et al. Effectiveness of an anesthetic continuous-infusion device in children with cerebral palsy undergoing orthopaedic surgery. J Pediatr Orthop 2010;30(8): 840–5.

51. Nowicki PD, Vanderhave KL, Gibbons K, et al. Perioperative pain control in pediatric patients undergoing orthopaedic surgery. J Am Acad Orthop Surg 2012;20(12):755–65.

52. Marzuillo P, Guarino S, Barbi E. Paracetamol: a focus for the general pediatrician. Eur J Pediatr 2014;173(4):415–25.

53. Sheehan WJ, Mauger DT, Paul IM, et al. Acetaminophen versus Ibuprofen in young children with mild persistent asthma. N Engl J Med 2016;375(7): 619–30.

54. Hiller A, Helenius I, Nurmi E, et al. Acetaminophen improves analgesia but does not reduce opioid requirement after major spine surgery in children and adolescents. Spine (Phila Pa 1976) 2012; 37(20):E1225–31.

55. Palmer GM. Pain management in the acute care setting: update and debates. J Paediatr Child Health 2016;52(2):213–20.

56. Wong I, St John-Green C, Walker SM. Opioid-sparing effects of perioperative paracetamol and nonsteroidal anti-inflammatory drugs (NSAIDs) in children. Paediatr Anaesth 2013;23(6):475–95.

57. Bhala N, Emberson J, Merhi A, et al. Vascular and upper gastrointestinal effects of non-steroidal anti-inflammatory drugs: meta-analyses of individual participant data from randomized trials. Lancet 2013;382:769–79.

58. Kay RM, Directo MP, Leathers M, et al. Complications of ketorolac use in children undergoing operative fracture care. J Pediatr Orthop 2010;30(7): 655–8.

59. Sucato DJ, Lovejoy JF, Agrawal S, et al. Postoperative ketorolac does not predispose to pseudoarthrosis following posterior spinal fusion and instrumentation for adolescent idiopathic scoliosis. Spine (Phila Pa 1976) 2008;33(10):1119–24.

60. Munro HM, Walton SR, Malviya S, et al. Low-dose ketorolac improves analgesia and reduces morphine requirements following posterior spinal fusion in adolescents. Can J Anaesth 2002;49(5): 461–6.

61. Rosenberg RE, Trzcinski S, Cohen M, et al. The association between adjuvant pain medication use and outcomes following pediatric spinal fusion. Spine (Phila Pa 1976) 2016;42:E602–8.

62. Rusy LM, Hainsworth KR, Nelson TJ, et al. Gabapentin use in pediatric spinal fusion patients: a randomized, double-blind, controlled trial. Anesth Analg 2010;110(5):1393–8.

63. Mayell A, Srinivasan I, Campbell F, et al. Analgesic effects of gabapentin after scoliosis surgery in children: a randomized controlled trial. Paediatr Anaesth 2014;24(12):1239–44.

64. Herring JA, editor. Tachdjian's pediatric orthopaedics. 3rd edition. Philadelphia: W. B. Saunders; 2001. p. 109–19.

65. Mycek MJ, Harvey RA, Chape PA, editors. Lippincott's illustrated reviews: pharmacology. 2nd edition. Philadelphia: Lippincott Williams & Wilkins; 2000.

66. U.S. Food and Drug Administration. FDA Drug Safety Communication: Safety review update of codeine use in children; new Boxed Warning and Contraindication on use after tonsillectomy and/or adenoidectomy. In: Drug Safety and Availability. 2013. Available at: https://www.fda.gov/Drugs/DrugSafety/ucm339112.htm. Accessed March 17, 2017.

67. Gasche Y, Daali Y, Fathi M, et al. Codeine intoxication associated with ultrarapid CYP2D6 metabolism. N Engl J Med 2004;351(27):2827–31.

68. Marco CA, Plewa MC, Buderer N, et al. Comparison of oxycodone and hydrocodone for the treatment of acute pain associated with fractures: a double-blind, randomized, controlled trial. Acad Emerg Med 2005;12(4):282–8.

69. Slawson D. No difference between oxycodone/acetaminophen and hydrocodone/acetaminophen for acute extremity pain. Am Fam Physician 2016; 93(5):411.

70. Grant DR, Schoenleber SJ, McCarthy AM, et al. Are we prescribing our patients too much pain medication? Best predictors of narcotic usage after spinal surgery for scoliosis. J Bone Joint Surg Am 2016; 98(18):1555–62.

71. Berde CB, Lehn BM, Yee JD, et al. Patient-controlled analgesia in children and adolescents: a randomized, prospective comparison with intramuscular administration of morphine for postoperative analgesia. J Pediatr 1991;118(3):460–6.

72. Monitto CL, Greenberg RS, Kost-Byerly S, et al. The safety and efficacy of parent-/nurse-controlled analgesia in patients less than six years of age. Anesth Analg 2000;91(3):573–9.

73. Muhly WT, Sankar WN, Ryan K, et al. Rapid recovery pathway after spinal fusion for idiopathic scoliosis. Pediatrics 2016;137(4) [pii:e20151568].

74. Eberson CP, Pacicca DM, Ehrlich MG. The role of ketorolac in decreasing length of stay and narcotic complications in the postoperative pediatric orthopaedic patient. J Pediatr Orthop 1999; 19(5):688–92.

75. Segal IS, Jarvis DJ, Duncan SR, et al. Clinical efficacy of oral-transdermal clonidine combinations during the perioperative period. Anesthesiology 1991;74(2):220–5.

76. Nota SP, Spit SA, Voskuyl T, et al. Opioid use, satisfaction, and pain intensity after orthopedic surgery. Psychosomatics 2015;56(5):479–85.

77. Connelly M, Fulmer RD, Prohaska J, et al. Predictors of postoperative pain trajectories in adolescent idiopathic scoliosis. Spine (Phila Pa 1976) 2014;39(3):E174–81.

78. Bot AG, Bekkers S, Arnstein PM, et al. Opioid use after fracture surgery correlates with pain intensity and satisfaction with pain relief. Clin Orthop Relat Res 2014;472(8):2542–9.

79. Davidson F, Snow S, Hayden JA, et al. Psychological interventions in managing postoperative pain in children: a systematic review. Pain 2016;157(9): 1872–86.

80. Swanson CE, Chang K, Schleyer E, et al. Postoperative pain control after supracondylar humerus fracture fixation. J Pediatr Orthop 2012;32(5): 452–5.

81. Georgopoulos G, Carry P, Pan Z, et al. The efficacy of intra-articular injections for pain control following the closed reduction and percutaneous pinning of pediatric supracondylar humeral fractures: a randomized controlled trial. J Bone Joint Surg Am 2012;94(18):1633–42.

82. Glover CD, Paek JS, Patel N, et al. Postoperative pain and the use of ultrasound-guided regional analgesia in pediatric supracondylar humerus fractures. J Pediatr Orthop B 2015;24(3):178–83.

83. Kucera TJ, Boezaart AP. Regional anesthesia does not consistently block ischemic pain: two further cases and a review of the literature. Pain Med 2014;15(2):316–9.

84. Brenn BR, Choudhry DK, Sacks K, et al. Toward better pain management: the development of a "Pain Stewardship Program" in a Tertiary Children's Hospital. Hosp Pediatr 2016;6(9):520–8.

85. Van Boerum DH, Smith JT, Curtin MJ. A comparison of the effects of patient-controlled analgesia with intravenous opioids versus Epidural analgesia on recovery after surgery for idiopathic scoliosis. Spine (Phila Pa 1976) 2000;25(18):2355–7.

86. Hong RA, Gibbons KM, Li GY, et al. A retrospective comparison of intrathecal morphine and epidural hydromorphone for analgesia following posterior spinal fusion in adolescents with idiopathic scoliosis. Paediatr Anaesth 2017;27(1):91–7.

Perioperative Pain Management in Pediatric Spine Surgery

Benjamin W. Sheffer, MD*, Derek M. Kelly, MD,
Leslie N. Rhodes, DNP, PPCNP/BC, Jeffrey R. Sawyer, MD

KEYWORDS

- Scoliosis • Pain management • Pediatric • Patient-controlled analgesia • Epidural

KEY POINTS

- Adequate pain control improves patient satisfaction and decreases hospital length of stay.
- Multimodal pain control helps provide adequate analgesia while minimizing adverse effects.
- Postoperative protocols, including pain management protocols, are important tools to help prepare nursing and other support staff to provide efficient and consistent care.

INTRODUCTION

Pain management after spinal deformity correction surgery for scoliosis in the pediatric population can be difficult due to the magnitude of the procedure. Deformity correction with posterior spinal fusion, with or without anterior procedures, causes significant tissue trauma that can result in debilitating pain. Historically, pain control has been achieved with intravenous (IV) opiates through patient-controlled anesthesia (PCA) or through IV push methods administered by nursing staff. Opiates provide excellent analgesic effect; however, the consequences of using opiates alone may include inadequate analgesia, nausea, vomiting, constipation, urinary retention, somnolence, respiratory depression, and possibly longer hospital stays, or even opiate dependence. In adult total joint arthroplasty, multimodal pain control has become an increasingly common method to achieve pain control without these sequelae. Recently, the same techniques have been studied in pediatric spinal deformity correction surgery as well. The purpose of this article is to outline the state of pain management in pediatric spine patients, including the use of multimodal management and to evaluate where further advances can be made.

OPIATES

Opiates are the mainstay of treatment for postoperative pain in many pediatric procedures, especially those in which the patient or surgeon expects significant postoperative pain. Opiates act on receptors in the brain, spinal cord, and peripheral tissues. There are several types of opiate-based pain medications that vary in their potency and duration of action. Opiates can be given in multiple different modalities including, but not limited to, orally, intravenously, by a patient-controlled anesthesia (PCA) device, an epidural injection, or intrathecal administration. Most patients are treated in the immediate postoperative period with IV or PCA methods and transitioned to oral-based intake, but adverse effects may limit the dose of opiates a patient can receive. Opiate administration also may prolong hospital stay if adverse effects require treatment or if the patient is unable to mobilize and participate in physical therapy. Despite this, opiates remain an effective analgesic, and they are used as the mainstay of treatment because of their potent analgesic properties. Tolerance to

Department of Orthopaedic Surgery and Biomedical Engineering, Campbell Clinic, The University of Tennessee Health Science Center, Le Bonheur Children's Hospital, 51 North Dunlap Street, Memphis, TN 38105, USA
* Corresponding author. 1400 S. Germantown Road, Germantown, TN 38138, USA.
E-mail address: bsheffer@campbellclinic.com

opiates can develop relatively quickly, with some medications more likely than others to cause this.

Acute opiate tolerance has been reported with the use of the medication remifentanil. Remifentanil is an opiate frequently used by anesthesia providers during spinal deformity surgery because of its potency, short duration of action, and lack of interference with neuromonitoring; however, it has been shown to cause acute opioid tolerance, leading to 30% higher opiate requirements in the postoperative period.[1] It is believed that opiate-related adverse events may be related to the total dose given. Minor adverse events, including vomiting, pruritus, and constipation, are common and occur in approximately 40%, 20% to 60%, and 15% to 90% of patients, respectively.[2] More severe adverse events such as respiratory depression occur much less frequently; in 1 review, the rate of respiratory depression was identified as 0.0013%.[2]

NONSTEROIDAL ANTI-INFLAMMATORY DRUGS

Nonsteroidal anti-inflammatory drugs (NSAIDs) are a group of medications whose primary mechanism of action is inhibition of the enzyme cyclooxygenase (COX). This leads to a decrease in the production of prostaglandins, which are involved in the inflammatory response. NSAIDs have been demonstrated to provide good analgesia while decreasing postoperative opiate use after posterior spinal fusion in pediatric scoliosis surgery.[3] This may lead to a decrease in opiate-related adverse effects. It has been shown that NSAIDs decrease the number of hospital days patients require PCA use and also decrease the likelihood of prolonged hospital length of stay, defined as 4 days or more in a scoliosis database review by Rosenberg.[4] The concern with the use of NSAIDs is that they have gastrointestinal (GI) and renal adverse effects and have been linked to delayed bone healing in animal models.[5] This has been corroborated in certain adult populations.[6] Sucato and colleagues[7] compared patients who received ketorolac and those who did not after posterior spinal fusion for adolescent idiopathic scoliosis. An overall pseudarthrosis rate of 2.5% was found, but ketorolac did not increase the likelihood of pseudarthrosis. There is also a concern about the effects of NSAIDs on platelet function by inhibiting formation of thromboxane A2; however, bleeding-related adverse events such as increased likelihood of transfusion or increased reoperation rates have not been associated with the use of ketorolac when given in the postoperative period.[8]

OTHER ANALGESICS

Acetaminophen

Acetaminophen is widely used for pain management, either alone or compounded with other medications such as opiates. Acetaminophen is commonly administered by mouth, intravenously, or rectally. IV acetaminophen has been shown to decrease visual analogue scale (VAS) pain scores in the first 24 hours after surgery for scoliosis; however, it has not been shown to decrease opiate requirements, and no patients in the study by Hiller and colleagues[9] reached toxic levels of acetaminophen. Caution must be used with acetaminophen whether orally or intravenously, because many commonly used oral pain medications are compounded with acetaminophen; the surgeon must be aware of total daily acetaminophen intake to avoid toxicity. The recommended maximal daily dose of acetaminophen in children is 75 mg/kg/d with hepatotoxicity occurring at 150 mg/kg/d. If dosages remain below toxic levels, acetaminophen has been shown to have an excellent adverse effect profile and is safe to use in this population.

Gabapentin

Gabapentin was synthesized to mimic the hormone gamma-aminobutyric acid (GABA), an inhibitory neurotransmitter in the central nervous system. It has been found to be useful in several medical conditions including epilepsy and migraines, as well as for pain control. Gabapentin has been shown to improve pain scores and decrease opiate consumption after total knee arthroplasty, hysterectomy, mastectomy, and certain adult spine surgeries.[10] It is thought that soft-tissue trauma may sensitize the sensory nerves, making them hyperexcitable postoperatively, and gabapentin may exert its effect by decreasing spontaneous sensory nerve firing. Gabapentin has been used in adolescent idiopathic scoliosis, and when given as a single dose of 600 mg preoperatively, leads to mixed results. Mayell and colleagues[10] randomized 35 patients into a group given a placebo and a group given 600 mg of gabapentin 1 hour before surgery. Although the patients who were given gabapentin required less morphine postoperatively, the results were not significantly different. However, when gabapentin is given preoperatively at a dose of 15 mg/kg and continued into the postoperative period at a dose of 5 mg/kg 3 times daily, it has been demonstrated to decrease opiate use on postoperative days 0, 1, and 2. Additionally, it was shown that pain scores were improved on postoperative day 0 and 1.[11] It appears that its effects of decreasing spontaneous sensory nerve firing wear off after postoperative day 2.

OTHER MEDICATIONS

Other medications have been used in treating postoperative pain after scoliosis surgery. Ketamine has been used in many ways, including a low-dose infusion for 72 hours; however, this did not affect pain scores or opiate consumption.[12] Benzodiazepines such as diazepam and muscle relaxants such as cyclobenzaprine frequently are given postoperatively to help with muscle spasm after surgery. Although there is little evidence to support their use, they are routinely given. Finally, local anesthetics such as lidocaine and bupivacaine can be placed around the surgical wound to help with local pain control or they may be used as part of a continuous infusion into the wound via a pump. One study showed that a continuous infusion of 0.25% bupivacaine at a rate of 4 mL/h decreased opiate use by 38% on postoperative day 1. After postoperative day 1, opiate use was similar.[13] However, the study did not compare continuous local anesthetic infusion to a single injection of local anesthetic to the wound at the time of closure.

REGIONAL ANESTHESIA

Epidural analgesia has been given in many forms for pain control after pediatric scoliosis surgery. An epidural provides excellent pain control and can be placed by the surgeon intraoperatively. It is important to note that local anesthetics used in the epidural regimen may make neurologic examination after surgery difficult and may mask an underlying neurologic injury. This can be avoided by dosing the epidural to start after completion of a detailed postoperative neurologic examination. Continuous epidural anesthesia has been shown to lead to improved pain scores[14] and decreased opiate use when compared with PCA, with decreased systemic side effects including nausea, constipation, and urinary retention.[15] An epidural catheter is even safe to use when the epidural space is exposed by Smith-Petersen osteotomies or when sublaminar cables are used.[16] Epidural catheters, however, have a relatively high failure rate of 8% to 37%.[14,17] Turner and colleagues[18] injected radiopaque dye into the epidural catheter before routine postoperative chest

radiographs were taken and found that 5 of 14 patients (35%) had inadequate pain control, and no dye was seen in the epidural space. Two of the 14 patients (14%) had dye in the paravertebral gutters, but had adequate pain control. The remaining patients had dye in the epidural space and had adequate pain control. The use of 2 catheters has been shown to decrease the failure rate and provide superior analgesia.[15] The epidural catheter has the potential to migrate in the spinal canal as well, with 32% migrating 1 segment and 8% migrating 2 segments.[19] The clinical significance of this is unknown, but if migration occurs outward, it may lead to inadequate analgesia. If the migration is inward, there is a potential for infection or neurologic injury; this was not observed in this study, which looked solely at migration.

Intrathecal administration of opiates is another option for regional anesthesia. This can be done preoperatively or by the surgeon directly injecting the dura. Intrathecal morphine has been shown to provide 12 to 36 hours of analgesia[20,21] and lead to decreased IV opiate requirements and improved pain scores compared with PCA.[20] There is also a correlation between intrathecal morphine use and decreased blood loss[21,22] in pediatric spinal fusion surgery for scoliosis. The exact mechanism is unknown, but it is thought to be related to a lower mean arterial pressure (MAP)[21]; however, another study showed an intrathecal dose-independent decrease in blood loss that was not associated with a lower MAP.[22] A concern with the use of intrathecal opiates is that the medication can migrate in the cerebrospinal fluid to the brainstem and potentially increase the risk of adverse effects. Although it has been shown that intrathecal opiates increase the risk of pruritus, as does epidural administration, other adverse effects such as nausea, vomiting, constipation, and respiratory depression are not increased with intrathecal opiates.[20,22,23] Intrathecal opiates are safe and provide a powerful adjunct for pain control in the first 12 to 36 hours after deformity correction surgery for scoliosis.

SUMMARY

Several options are available to help alleviate pain after deformity correction surgery for scoliosis in the pediatric patient (Table 1). A multimodal approach to pain control provides superior analgesia while minimizing adverse effects. The patient's experience with pain and pain control is important in the patient's perception of outcome. Postoperative protocols that

Table 1
Pain management options after spinal deformity correction surgery for scoliosis in the pediatric patient

Medication	Mechanism of Action	Administration	Adverse Effects	Notes
Opioid analgesics • Morphine • Hydromorphone • Fentanyl • Meperidine • Oxycodone • Hydrocodone • Codeine	• Bind mu, kappa, delta opioid receptors in central nervous system (CNS) and peripherally • Inhibit transmission of nociceptive stimuli • Activate descending inhibitory pathways to the spinal cord • Alter limbic system pathways to change emotional and behavioral response to pain	• By mouth • Rectally • Transdermal • Intramuscular • Intravenously • PCA • Epidural • Intrathecal	• Nausea • Vomiting • Constipation • Pruritus • Urinary retention • Sedation • Confusion • Respiratory depression	• Overdose treated with naloxone • May need repeat treatment as effects last up to 1 h
NSAIDs • Ketorolac • Ibuprofen • Naproxen • Meloxicam • Diclofenac • Other	• Inhibition of COX, preventing synthesis of prostaglandins	• By mouth • Intravenously	• GI-ulcers • Bleeding-antiplatelet function by blocking platelet aggregation • Acute kidney injury	• Ketorolac use should not exceed 5 d.
Acetaminophen	• Not well defined, possibly CNS COX inhibition • Modulation of endogenous cannabinoid system	• By mouth • Rectally • Intravenously	• Liver toxicity	• Maximal daily dose of 75 mg/kg • Caution in patients with liver disease • Lacks anti-inflammatory effects of NSAIDs
Gabapentin	• Not well defined, possibly binding voltage gated calcium channels of sensory nerves preventing pain transmission	• By mouth	• Fatigue • Dizziness • Somnolence	• Dosing varies. 15 mg/kg once preoperatively, then 5 mg/kg 3 times daily postoperatively while inpatient

include pain protocols have been shown to improve patient satisfaction and pain scores.[24] Accelerated pathways that admit the patient to the floor after surgery, rather than to the intensive care unit, have been shown to decrease the cost of care by about $5000 per patient[25,26] and require multimodal pain management to be successful. Adequate pain control is essential to help patients mobilize, improve patient satisfaction, and decrease patient and family stress postoperatively.

REFERENCES

1. Crawford MW, Hickey C, Zaarour C, et al. Development of acute opioid tolerance during infusion of remifentanil for pediatric scoliosis surgery. Anesth Analg 2006;102(6):1662–7.

2. Jitpakdee T, Mandee S. Strategies for preventing side effects of systemic opioid in postoperative pediatric patients. Paediatr Anaesth 2014;24: 561–8.

3. Munro HM, Walton SR, Malviya S, et al. Low-dose ketorolac improves analgesia and reduces morphine requirements following posterior spinal fusion in adolescents. Can J Anaesth 2002;49(5): 461–6.

4. Rosenberg RE, Trzcinski S, Cohen M, et al. The association between adjuvant pain medication use and outcomes following pediatric spinal fusion. Spine (Phila Pa 1976) 2016;42(10):E602–8.

5. Keller J, Bunger C, Andreassen TT, et al. Bone repair inhibited by indomethacin. Effects on bone metabolism and strength of rabbit osteotomies. Acta Orthop Scand 1987;58:379–83.

6. Glassman SD, Rose SM, Dimar JR, et al. The effect of postoperative nonsteroidal anti-inflammatory drug administration on spinal fusion. Spine 1998; 23:834–8.

7. Sucato DJ, Lovejoy JF, Agrawal S, et al. Postoperative ketorolac does not predispose to pseudoarthrosis following posterior spinal fusion and instrumentation for adolescent idiopathic scoliosis. Spine (Phila Pa 1976) 2008;33(10):1119–24.

8. Vitale MG, Choe JC, Hwang MW, et al. Use of ketorolac tromethamine in children undergoing scoliosis surgery. An analysis of complications. Spine J 2003;3(1):55–62.

9. Hiller A, Helenius I, Nurmi E, et al. Acetaminophen improves analgesia but does not reduce opioid requirement after major spine surgery in children and adolescents. Spine (Phila Pa 1976) 2012; 37(20):E1225–31.

10. Mayell A, Srinivasan I, Campbell F, et al. Analgesic effects of gabapentin after scoliosis surgery in children: a randomized controlled trial. Paediatr Anaesth 2014;24(12):1239–44.

11. Rusy LM, Hainsworth KR, Nelson TJ, et al. Gabapentin use in pediatric spinal fusion patients: a randomized, double-blind, controlled trial. Anesth Analg 2010;110(5):1393–8.

12. Pestieau SR, Finkel JC, Junqueira MM, et al. Prolonged perioperative infusion of low-dose ketamine does not alter opioid use after pediatric scoliosis surgery. Paediatr Anaesth 2014;24(6): 582–90.

13. Reynolds RA, Legakis JE, Tweedie J, et al. Postoperative pain management after spinal fusion surgery: an analysis of the efficacy of continuous infusion of local anesthetics. Global Spine J 2013; 3(1):7–14.

14. Sucato DJ, Duey-Holtz A, Elerson E, et al. Postoperative analgesia following surgical correction for adolescent idiopathic scoliosis: a comparison of continuous epidural analgesia and patient-controlled analgesia. Spine (Phila Pa 1976) 2005; 30(2):211–7.

15. Klatt JW, Mickelson J, Hung M, et al. A randomized prospective evaluation of 3 techniques of postoperative pain management after posterior spinal instrumentation and fusion. Spine (Phila Pa 1976) 2013;38(19):1626–31.

16. Lavelle ED, Lavelle WF, Goodwin R, et al. Epidural analgesia for postoperative pain control after adolescent spinal fusion procedures which violated the epidural space. J Spinal Disord Tech 2010;23(5): 347–50.

17. Gauger VT, Voepel-Lewis TD, Burke CN, et al. Epidural analgesia compared with intravenous analgesia after pediatric posterior spinal fusion. J Pediatr Orthop 2009;29(6):588–93.

18. Turner A, Lee J, Mitchell R, et al. The efficacy of surgically placed epidural catheters for analgesia after posterior spinal surgery. Anaesthesia 2000;55: 370–3.

19. Strandness T, Wiktor M, Varadarajan J, et al. Migration of pediatric epidural catheters. Paediatr Anaesth 2015;25(6):610–3.

20. Milbrandt TA, Singhal M, Minter C, et al. A comparison of three methods of pain control for posterior spinal fusions in adolescent idiopathic scoliosis. Spine (Phila Pa 1976) 2009;34(14):1499–503.

21. Dalens B, Tanguy A. Intrathecal morphine for spinal fusion in children. Spine (Phila Pa 1976) 1988;13(5): 494–8.

22. Eschertzhuber S, Hohlrieder M, Keller C, et al. Comparison of high- and low-dose intrathecal morphine for spinal fusion in children. Br J Anaesth 2008;100(4):538–43.

23. Yen D, Turner K, Mark D. Is a single low dose of intrathecal morphine a useful adjunct to patient-controlled analgesia for postoperative pain control following lumbar spine surgery? A preliminary report. Pain Res Manag 2015;20(3):129–32.

24. Rao RR, Hayes M, Lewis C, et al. Mapping the road to recovery: shorter stays and satisfied patients in posterior spinal fusion. J Pediatr Orthop 2016. [Epub ahead of print].

25. Sanders A, Andras L, Sousa T, et al. Accelerated discharge protocol for posterior spinal fusion (PSF) patients with adolescent idiopathic scoliosis (AIS) decreases hospital post-operative charges 22%. Spine (Phila Pa 1976) 2017. 42L92–7.

26. Available at: http://americanpainsociety.org/uploads/education/section_3.pdf. Accessed April 19, 2017.

Upper Extremity

Perioperative Pain Management for Upper Extremity Surgery

Alexander C. Coleman, MD

KEYWORDS

- Anesthesia • Upper extremity • Wide-awake local anesthesia
- Local anesthesia with intravenous sedation • Intravenous regional block

KEY POINTS

- Anesthesia options range from general anesthesia to wide-awake local anesthesia.
- Anesthesia choice must be individualized for each patient.
- Patient factors to be considered include disease process and comorbidities.
- Procedure-related factors to consider include anatomic location and complexity and duration of the procedure, as well as postoperative pain expectations.

HISTORY OF UPPER EXTREMITY ANESTHESIA

The past 2 centuries have seen the rapid growth of effective pain control during and after upper extremity surgery. During the mid–eighteenth century, the happy coincidence of Dr Morton's introduction of ether as a general anesthetic and Dr Fergusson's development of the open palmar fasciectomy allowed what was likely the first hand surgery ever performed under general anesthesia.[1] This groundbreaking procedure occurred in 1846 and the advances in perioperative pain management have continued to this day.

Upper extremity surgeons are now faced with a daunting array of anesthesia techniques, ranging from traditional general anesthetic to wide-awake surgery, during which patients can watch their surgeons operate in the morning and return to work as soon as that afternoon. Because of this range of options, surgeons must develop an algorithm that sorts patients by disease process, relevant comorbidities, and procedure type to ensure each patient receives the most appropriate anesthetic option.

ANESTHESIA SELECTION

As a general rule, at our institution, the approach to upper extremity anesthesia care is to use local anesthesia if possible, and general anesthesia if necessary. The algorithm is simple. Surgeons assess the procedure and try to determine the least invasive anesthesia technique possible. There are multiple factors that go into this process:

1. What is the overall health status of the patient and what type of anesthesia will the patient tolerate?
2. What are the anatomic considerations of the procedure and what interventions will be needed to totally anesthetize that body part?
3. What is the duration of the procedure and will a tourniquet be required?
4. How painful will the procedure be, and what is the plan for postprocedure pain control?

Answering these basic questions aids surgeons in selecting the most effective and least invasive technique possible. It is also helpful to create broad anesthesia categories and then stratify them by invasiveness and relative risk to the patient. These categories are listed here in

Disclosures: None.
Andrews Institute for Orthopaedics & Sports Medicine, 1040 Gulf Breeze Pky, #200, Gulf Breeze, FL 32561, USA
E-mail address: colemanac@gmail.com

Orthop Clin N Am 48 (2017) 487–494
http://dx.doi.org/10.1016/j.ocl.2017.06.009
0030-5898/17/© 2017 Elsevier Inc. All rights reserved.

order of increasing invasiveness or anesthetic risk:

- Wide-awake local (no sedation)
- Local with intravenous (IV) sedation (local and monitored anesthesia care [MAC])
- IV regional (Bier block)
- Regional block (plexus block)
- General anesthesia

Local Only

In 1884, the German ophthalmologist Carl Koller discovered that, when he placed cocaine on his tongue, it quickly went numb.[2] He rapidly made the connection between drug and effect and introduced the use of cocaine as a local anesthetic to the practice of medicine. This development, inauspicious as it may seem with the benefit of hindsight, signaled the dawn of the era of modern anesthesia. Novocaine was discovered in 1905 and soon thereafter epinephrine was added to the armamentarium.

Local-only anesthesia is typically achieved by infiltration of an anesthetic agent at or near the site of a surgical procedure. This anesthesia can be accomplished either through a field block or by anesthetizing the nerves that service the surgical site. Two of the most common applications are local infiltration for trigger finger release or a digital nerve block for nail bed repair.

Local anesthesia has the advantage of avoiding any sedatives or narcotics. This advantage makes it attractive for patients with medical comorbidities or contraindications to anesthesia. It is also attractive to busy patients who do not want to take time off from work or who wish to drive themselves to and from the procedure. Disadvantages include pain associated with the injection, lack of sedatives for nervous patients, and the inability to use a forearm or arm tourniquet for more than 20 to 30 minutes. Another potential disadvantage of local infiltration is the presence of additional fluid at the surgical site, which can distort the anatomy and make visualization of critical structures more challenging.

Local with Intravenous Sedation

Many of the disadvantages of local-only anesthesia can be mediated through the judicious administration of IV sedatives and analgesics. Local anesthesia with sedation, or local MAC, provides a good balance of patient comfort, operative flexibility, and anesthetic risk. Although sometimes performed in the office setting, most orthopedists prefer to use this type of anesthesia in the operating room or ambulatory surgery center setting under the supervision of an anesthesiologist or certified registered nurse anesthetist. The addition of sedation has several distinct advantages. It provides comfort for anxious patients, helps alleviate the discomfort associated with anesthetic injection, and typically allows a longer tourniquet time. The level of sedation can also be incrementally increased if the patient is not tolerating the procedure. The primary drawbacks include the need for additional personnel in the form of an anesthesia team, increased cardiopulmonary risk and postoperative nausea, and the need for a caretaker to drive the patient home and observe the patient after surgery.

Intravenous Regional Anesthesia

German surgeon August Bier first described the use of IV regional anesthesia in 1908, but it did not gain widespread popularity until it was reintroduced in 1968 by Holmes.[3] The concept is simple. The operative extremity is completely exsanguinated and a tourniquet is inflated. The venous system is then back-filled with a large volume of local anesthetic, which diffuses throughout the distal extremity producing effective regional anesthesia. In the past, a double tourniquet was used over the brachium to allow longer tourniquet times by allowing for an additional site of tourniquet compression during the procedure. The primary disadvantage of this technique is the volume of anesthetic and the time required to administer the block, both of which can lead to delays in turnover. If a tourniquet is deflated prematurely, the large volume of anesthetic required for a Bier block can cause systemic toxicity.

At our institution, Bier block anesthesia is used on a routine basis. We overcome the problems mentioned earlier with the following modifications. First, the IV line for the block is placed in preoperative holding to save operating room time. We have also shifted to the use of a single-bladder forearm tourniquet with a significantly reduced volume of local anesthetic, thus allowing safe deflation of the tourniquet at any time during the procedure. Regardless of technique, IV regional anesthesia requires the use of a tourniquet in an awake or mildly sedated patient and thus can only be used for limited duration because of tourniquet pain. For this reason, it is best reserved for shorter procedures.

Regional Anesthesia (Plexus Blocks)

German surgeon Diedrich Kulenkampff is credited with performing the first percutaneous brachial plexus block in 1911.[4] He reportedly performed the first block on himself, and subsequently described 25 consecutive blocks with an 80% success rate. By 1928, brachial plexus anesthesia was rapidly becoming an established technique, with more than 1000 published procedures with an 80% success rate and a complication rate of 3%.[5] Although the use of electrical nerve stimulation was first described only a year after Kulenkampff's first block, early equipment was cumbersome and unreliable. Until the 1960s, plexus localization was achieved primarily by anatomic landmarks and eliciting paresthesias with the needle tip. In 1962, the first portable, reliable electronic nerve stimulator was introduced and quickly became the mainstay of localization until the introduction of ultrasonography in the 1980s. Since its introduction, the quality and portability of ultrasonography equipment has improved dramatically, and it has become the gold standard for nerve localization in brachial plexus blocks.

General Anesthesia

As the availability and effectiveness of regional anesthetic techniques has steadily increased, the use of general anesthesia in upper extremity surgery has been declining.[6] However, there is still a significant role for general anesthesia. Prime examples are patients with polytrauma who need multiple simultaneous procedures, children who do not hold still with sedation, and patients with contraindications to a regional block. Other cases may involve patients with ineffective blocks or those who refuse them.

ANESTHESIA TECHNIQUES

Local Anesthesia and Hand Surgery

Most procedures involving the hand and fingers can be safely and comfortably performed under local anesthesia.[7] There are many accepted techniques, each with its own advantages and drawbacks. The most common techniques are distal nerve blocks (wrist block or digital block), field blocks (local infiltration anesthesia), and local area blocks (tumescent local anesthesia).

Distal Peripheral Nerve Blocks

Distal nerve blocks at the wrist or digital level are effective for a wide range of hand procedures. Distal blocks have several distinct advantages:

- They can be comfortably performed with or without sedation.[8]
- They can provide 10 to 15 hours of anesthetic effect.[9]
- They do not introduce excess fluid into the operative field.

The primary disadvantage of a distal nerve block is that, even with the use of epinephrine-containing anesthetic, it does not provide hemostasis and may even cause distal vasodilation,[8] necessitating the use of a tourniquet. For procedures of the distal digit this can be mitigated by using a digital tourniquet; however, for more proximal work in the digit and palm, a forearm tourniquet may be required, which in turn may limit the duration of the procedure because of tourniquet intolerance.

Wrist blocks

Wrist blocks provide effective anesthesia for a wide range of hand procedures. The primary advantage compared with more proximal blocks is the sparing of the extrinsic muscles of the forearm, which allows active intraoperative digital motion. Depending on the location of the surgical site, the surgeon may need to anesthetize 1 or more of the 3 major peripheral nerves supplying the hand.

Median nerve block. The median nerve is located in the interval between the palmaris longus and flexor carpi radialis tendons. Green and Wolfe[10] described a safe method of blocking the median nerve at the wrist by injecting 5 to 7 mL of local anesthetic just ulnar to the palmaris longus tendon. The trajectory is at a 30° angle to the skin, aiming in a slightly radial direction to enter the carpal tunnel (**Fig. 1**). Clinicians should avoid eliciting paresthesias because this may indicate injury to the nerve. This technique can also be used for therapeutic carpal tunnel injections.

Ulnar nerve block. The ulnar nerve traverses the wrist between the ulnar artery and the flexor carpi ulnaris (FCU) tendon. The ulnar nerve can be blocked at this location by flexing the wrist

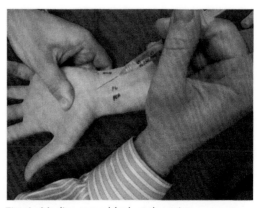

Fig. 1. Median nerve block at the wrist.

to allow visualization of the FCU tendon and injecting 5 mL of anesthetic just radial to the tendon (**Figs. 2** and **3**).[10] It is important to avoid eliciting paresthesias and to aspirate to confirm that an intra-arterial injection does not occur. It is also important to note that the dorsal ulnar cutaneous nerve branches 8 cm above the wrist crease and thus must be blocked separately to provide complete anesthesia to the ulnar aspect of the hand. This block can be accomplished by injecting a subcutaneous wheal of anesthesia from the ulnar aspect of the FCU extending dorsally to the fifth compartment.

Superficial radial nerve block. The superficial radial nerve travels in the subcutaneous tissues directly over the radial styloid. The nerve can be blocked in this location by subcutaneous infiltration of local anesthetic from just radial to the artery around the radial aspect of the wrist to the dorsal midline (**Fig. 4**).

Digital blocks
Blocking the digital nerves at the base of the finger or distal to the carpal tunnel in the palm provides effective long-lasting anesthesia for 1 or more digits. These techniques are safe and simple. The classic technique uses paired dorsal injections on either side of the digit. The theory behind this is that the dorsal skin is less sensitive so the injection is less painful. There is now level I and level II evidence to discredit that theory and propose that a single volar injection is better tolerated than paired dorsal injections.[11] The author has found this to be true in practice and has abandoned the classic 2-injection technique in favor of a single volar injection.

Digital block technique. The common digital nerves exit the carpal tunnel and divide into the proper digital nerves in the palm. The neurovascular bundles run on either side of the

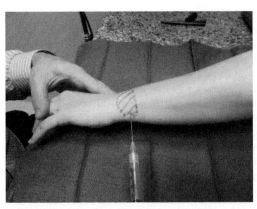

Fig. 3. Dorsal ulnar cutaneous nerve block.

flexor tendon sheaths deep to the palmar fascia. They enter the digit in a volar ulnar and volar radial position. At the level of the proximal phalanx they give off branches to supply the dorsal finger distal to the proximal interphalangeal (PIP) joint. Lalonde and Martin[8] described the SIMPLE[12] (single injection in the midline of the proximal phalanx with lidocaine with epinephrine) technique of digital block anesthesia: a single injection with a small volume of anesthetic (2 mL) (**Figs. 5** and **6**). This technique provides adequate anesthesia for the entire volar finger and the dorsal digit distal to the PIP joint. If more proximal anesthesia is required dorsally, a supplemental small-volume injection can be placed over the dorsum of the proximal phalanx, thus providing complete digital anesthesia. Note that the epinephrine provides hemostasis only around the injection site. Procedures distal to the PIP flexion crease require a digital tourniquet for hemostasis. In patients with relative contraindications to the use of epinephrine-containing anesthetic, plain lidocaine or bupivacaine hydrochloride can be used with the application of a digital tourniquet.

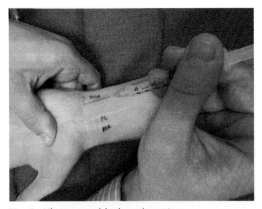

Fig. 2. Ulnar nerve block at the wrist.

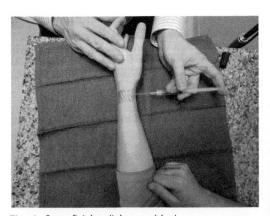

Fig. 4. Superficial radial nerve block.

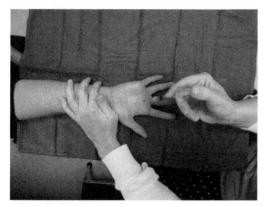

Fig. 5. Digital nerve block in the palm.

At our institution, we perform digital block anesthesia by injecting 10 mL of anesthetic just proximal to the palmar digital crease superficial to the A1 pulley. We typically use a mixture of plain xylocaine and bupivacaine buffered with 1 mL of sodium bicarbonate. The needle is introduced perpendicular to the skin and 1 to 2 mL is injected followed by a 30-second pause to allow the injection pain to resolve. Injection of the remaining anesthetic is typically painless. If it is necessary to work on the proximal dorsal aspect of the digit, the volar injection is supplemented by 2 to 3 mL of anesthetic injected dorsally just proximal to the metacarpophalangeal joint. This technique provides long-lasting anesthesia to the entire digit and allows dissection proximally to the midpalm.

Tumescent local anesthesia using lidocaine with epinephrine

Wide-awake local anesthesia with no tourniquet (WALANT) has seen a significant increase in popularity over the past decade. Dr Lalonde deserves much of the credit for this trend. Although there were many great hand surgeons

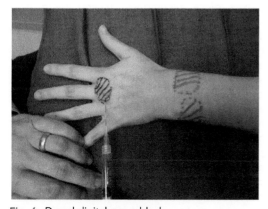

Fig. 6. Dorsal digital nerve block.

using this technique previously, Dr Lalonde has brought it to the forefront through his excellent research on the use of epinephrine-containing anesthetics in hand surgery. The concept is simple. Tourniquet pain is the primary obstacle to pure local anesthesia in hand surgery. WALANT does away with the tourniquet by using the vasoconstrictive properties of epinephrine. No tourniquet means no tourniquet pain, which in turn translates to no sedatives or narcotic analgesia during the procedure. This process greatly simplifies the perioperative period. No sedative means fewer personnel, less medical risk, and no need for a driver or postoperative caretaker. This simplification reduces cost and improves efficiency and convenience. It also means the patient is fully awake and cooperative during the procedure. The patient can show active motion during the procedure, allowing the surgeons to fine-tune their work. Patients also see what is being done and what they are capable of doing with the affected extremity, which can serve as positive reinforcement during rehabilitation.

The primary barrier to WALANT anesthesia is the fear of epinephrine. All medical students are taught never to inject epinephrine into fingers, toes, nose, or hose. The surprising fact is that there is little evidence to support this mantra. In a 2007 literature review, Thomson and colleagues[13] reviewed the evidence for and against epinephrine use in the fingers and found little to no support for the paradigm. In 2005, Lalonde and colleagues[14] published the results of the Dalhousie Project, a multicenter study involving 9 hand surgeons. They performed 3110 consecutive hand procedures using lidocaine containing epinephrine with no instances of digital necrosis and no cases in which phentolamine rescue was required.[14] There have been a multitude of follow-up studies showing the safe and efficacious use of epinephrine in the hand.[15] Although all of this evidence suggests that the myth is debunked and that epinephrine is safe to use in the hand, there have been 2 recent case reports of digital ischemia following epinephrine injection in the hand.[16,17] Both reports involved ischemia of digits following epinephrine injection for trigger finger surgery in patients without known vasoconstrictive disease. In one of the cases, phentolamine rescue was performed and the ischemia was reversed without any tissue necrosis.[16] In the other case, rescue was not performed and fingertip necrosis occurred.[17] Although these represent only 2 ischemic events out of many thousands of injections, they nonetheless suggest the potential need for phentolamine rescue, so surgeons using WALANT should be prepared for that possibility.

Phentolamine rescue. Phentolamine is an alpha-adrenergic blocker that has been proved to reverse the effects of epinephrine injection in the finger.[18] Phentolamine is widely available and can be used to reverse the effects of epinephrine by injecting it into the area where epinephrine was previously injected. In a randomized trial comparing phentolamine injection with saline, Nodwell and Lalonde[18] showed that injection of 1 mg of phentolamine and 1 mL of saline directly into the site of the previous injection reversed the effects of epinephrine at an average time of 85 minutes.

Tumescent local anesthesia technique. Tumescent local anesthesia uses large volumes of epinephrine-containing local anesthetic to provide both analgesia and hemostasis during the operative procedure. The surgical area is injected with anesthetic, typically lidocaine with 1:100,000 epinephrine, until the skin becomes tumescent and blanched by the vasoconstrictive effects of the epinephrine. The area of blanched skin should extend at least 1 cm beyond all proposed incision sites.[8] It takes an average of 26 minutes to reach the optimal vasoconstrictive effects of epinephrine, and thus the injection should be performed 30 minutes before the start of the procedure.[19] In the ambulatory surgery center setting, this can be achieved by injecting the patient in the preoperative holding area. For in-office procedures, the patient can return to the waiting area following injection to allow for local anesthetic to set up. If appropriately timed and orchestrated, this technique can allow multiple consecutive procedures to be performed with minimal turnover time between patients. Dr Lalonde's[8] book *Wide Awake Hand Surgery* provides in-depth discussion of WALANT. He covers both the technical aspects of the various injection techniques as well as methods to improve efficiency and convenience for both surgeons and patients. The text is informative and well organized, and it is highly recommended to anyone considering expanding their WALANT practice.

Brachial Plexus Blocks

The number and complexity of upper extremity cases being performed in an outpatient setting have seen dramatic increases in recent decades.[20] This trend is in large part a product of advances in regional anesthesia techniques. In particular the brachial plexus blockade has allowed complex upper extremity surgery without the use of general anesthesia.[21] A single-shot brachial plexus block can provide effective anesthesia and analgesia for the duration of the procedure and 12 to 24 hours postoperatively. The addition of continuous blockade catheters has allowed effective pain control well into the early postoperative period.

Although it is beyond the scope of this article to address the technical aspects of each type of brachial plexus block, it is useful for surgeons to possess a basic working knowledge of the main types of blocks and the procedures for which they are most effective. There are 4 major types of plexus blocks that encompass most upper extremity regional anesthesia: (1) the interscalene block, (2) the supraclavicular block, (3) infraclavicular blocks, and (4) the axillary block.

Interscalene block

The interscalene block provides anesthesia to the proximal upper extremity by targeting the trunks of the brachial plexus in the groove between the anterior and middle scalene muscles. The interscalene block provides good coverage of the entire shoulder as well as the radial aspect of the arm. It has limited coverage of the medial arm, elbow, and hand. The interscalene block is the workhorse of shoulder surgery. It has the advantage of being technically easier in obese patients, and it can be performed in any arm position, making it a good choice for proximal humerus fractures. It also has a lower reported risk of pneumothorax.[22] Known complications include Horner syndrome, hemidiaphragm paralysis, and hoarseness.[23] In addition, the anatomy of the interscalene region allows secure placement of a continuous nerve block catheter and is therefore a good choice for cases in which ambulatory continuous regional anesthesia is desired.

Supraclavicular block

The supraclavicular block is the oldest of the plexus block techniques, having been first described by Kulenkampff in 1911.[24] The supraclavicular block targets the trunks of the entire plexus where they are most tightly packaged in a fascial sheath, which includes the subclavian artery. The supraclavicular technique provides complete blockade of the entire plexus, giving excellent anesthesia to the entire distal two-thirds of the extremity. It is well suited to surgery from the midhumerus to the hand and provides sufficient anesthesia for an upper arm tourniquet. It is not ideally suited for continuous catheter placement because of anatomic constraints. The supraclavicular technique places the needle in close proximity to the cupula of the lung, which increases the risk of pneumothorax. In a prospective study of more than 6000 periclavicular blocks, Gauss and colleagues[25] showed that the use of ultrasonography guidance can reduce that risk to 0.06%.

Infraclavicular block

The infraclavicular block targets the cords of the plexus where they reside in the axillary sheath deep into the clavicle. The supraclavicular block provides reliable anesthesia from the elbow to the hand. It also reliably blocks the axillary and musculocutaneous nerves and allows the use of an upper arm tourniquet. The anatomy of the region facilitates the placement of a continuous catheter and thus is ideal for cases in which ambulatory continuous nerve blockade is desired. The risk of pneumothorax is reduced compared with the supraclavicular approach because of a more favorable trajectory of the needle relative to the lung.

Axillary block

The axillary block targets the terminal branches of the plexus at the level of the distal axillary sheath. The axillary nerve is not affected at this level and the musculocutaneous nerve is often outside of the sheath, necessitating special attention. The axillary block provides excellent anesthesia distal to the elbow. Because it is far removed from the critical structures of the neck, the safety profile is excellent, especially when ultrasonography guidance is used.[26] However, because of anatomic constraints, the axillary block is not well suited to the placement of a continuous catheter.

FUTURE DIRECTIONS

The ideal anesthetic is safe, effective, and long lasting. Key features would include minimal risk in both the administration of the anesthetic and its effect on comorbid conditions. There would be minimal discomfort during administration of the anesthetic and minimal side effects afterward. The anesthetic should provide complete analgesia during the procedure. In addition, it should have a long postoperative duration to minimize the need for narcotics during the early postoperative period.

Improvements in regional blockade techniques, including the use of continuous catheters, have achieved many of these goals; however, there is still the risk of block-related complications, including the potential failure of continuous blockade catheters. A potential solution to these problems may have arrived in

the form of extended-duration local anesthetics. Liposomal bupivacaine, sold under the trade name Exparel, seeks to fulfill that role. Although there are promising early data in arthroplasty, there are minimal data as yet to support its use in hand surgery. At the time of this publication, a literature search for Exparel and hand surgery yielded a single article comparing the use of lidocaine, Marcaine, and Exparel in trigger finger surgery.[27] The study's results were promising, but more work needs to be done before this can become the standard of care. In theory, a single shot of an extended local anesthetic either at the plexus level or the distal peripheral nerve level could provide long-lasting analgesia well into the early postoperative period without the added risk and encumbrance of a continuous peripheral nerve catheter. As the country faces an ever-growing opioid epidemic, the need for safe, effective, opioid-sparing anesthesia techniques has never been greater.

REFERENCES

1. Petermann H. Crawford Williamson Long - The true discoverer of anesthesia? Anasthesiol Intensivmed Notfallmed Schmerzther 2016;51(10):636–9 [in German].
2. Goerig M. From the legacy of Carl Koller. Notations on his experiments with cocaine. Anaesthesist 2015;64(6):469–77 [in German].
3. dos Reis A Jr. Intravenous regional anesthesia–first century (1908-2008). Beggining, development, and current status [review]. Rev Bras Anestesiol 2008; 58(3):299–321 [in English, Portuguese].
4. Livingston EM. Brachial plexus block: its clinical application. Address to joint meeting, American Society of Regional Anesthesia: Canadian Society of Anesthetists: Eastern Society of Anesthetists. Montreal, Canada, October 27, 1926.
5. Kulenkampff D. Brachial plexus anaesthesia: its indications, technique, and dangers. Ann Surg 1928;87(6):883–91.
6. Patel AA, Buller LT, Fleming ME, et al. National trends in ambulatory surgery for upper extremity fractures: a 10-year analysis of the US National Survey of Ambulatory Surgery. Hand (N Y) 2015;10(2): 254–9.
7. Lalonde D, Eaton C, Amadio P, et al. Wide-awake hand and wrist surgery: a new horizon in outpatient surgery [review]. Instr Course Lect 2015;64:249–59.
8. Lalonde DH. Wide awake hand surgery. New York: Thieme Medical Publishers; 2011.
9. Calder K, Chung B, O'Brien C, et al. Bupivacaine digital blocks: how long is the pain relief and

temperature elevation? Plast Reconstr Surg 2013; 131(5):1098–104.

10. Green D, Wolfe S. Green's operative hand surgery. Philadelphia: Elsevier/Churchill Livingstone; 2011.

11. Williams JG. Randomized comparison of the single-injection volar subcutaneous block and the two-injection dorsal block for digital anesthesia. Plast Reconstr Surg 2006;118(5):1195–200.

12. Wheelock ME, Leblanc M, Chung B, et al. Is it true that injecting palmar finger skin hurts more than dorsal skin? New level 1 evidence. Hand (N Y) 2011;6(1):47–9.

13. Thomson CJ, Lalonde DH, Denkler KA, et al. A critical look at the evidence for and against elective epinephrine use in the finger [review]. Plast Reconstr Surg 2007;119(1):260–6.

14. Lalonde D, Bell M, Benoit P, et al. A multicenter prospective study of 3,110 consecutive cases of elective epinephrine use in the fingers and hand: the Dalhousie Project clinical phase. J Hand Surg Am 2005;30(5):1061–7.

15. Hagert E, Lalonde D. Time to bury the adrenaline-myth!–Safe use of adrenaline anesthesia in hand surgery and orthopedics [review]. Lakartidningen 2015;112 [in Swedish].

16. Zhu AF, Hood BR, Morris MS, et al. Delayed-onset digital ischemia after local anesthetic with epinephrine injection requiring phentolamine reversal. J Hand Surg Am 2017;42(6):479.e1–4.

17. Zhang JX, Gray J, Lalonde DH, et al. Digital necrosis after lidocaine and epinephrine injection in the flexor tendon sheath without phentolamine rescue. J Hand Surg Am 2017;42(2):e119–23.

18. Nodwell T, Lalonde D. How long does it take phentolamine to reverse adrenaline-induced vasoconstriction in the finger and hand? A prospective, randomized, blinded study: the Dalhousie Project experimental phase. Can J Plast Surg 2003;11(4): 187–90.

19. Mckee DE, Lalonde DH, Thoma A, et al. Achieving the optimal epinephrine effect in wide awake hand surgery using local anesthesia without a tourniquet. Hand (N Y) 2015;10(4):613–5.

20. Pregler JL, Kapur PA. The development of ambulatory anesthesia and future challenges. Anesthesiol Clin North America 2003;21(2):207–28.

21. Srikumaran U, Stein BE, Tan EW, et al. Upper-extremity peripheral nerve blocks in the perioperative pain management of orthopaedic patients: AAOS exhibit selection [review]. J Bone Joint Surg Am 2013;95(24):e197(1-13).

22. Mian A, Chaudhry I, Huang R, et al. Brachial plexus anesthesia: a review of the relevant anatomy, complications, and anatomical variations [review]. Clin Anat 2014;27(2):210–21.

23. Beal MF. Neuroprotective effects of creatine [review]. Amino Acids 2011;40(5):1305–13.

24. Lalonde D, Martin A. Epinephrine in local anesthesia in finger and hand surgery: the case for wide-awake anesthesia. J Am Acad Orthop Surg 2013;21(8):443–7.

25. Gauss A, Tugtekin I, Georgieff M, et al. Incidence of clinically symptomatic pneumothorax in ultrasound-guided infraclavicular and supraclavicular brachial plexus block. Anaesthesia 2014;69(4):327–36.

26. Satapathy AR, Coventry DM. Axillary brachial plexus block. Anesthesiol Res Pract 2011;2011: 173796.

27. Ketonis C, Kim N, Liss F, et al. Wide awake trigger finger release surgery: prospective comparison of lidocaine, Marcaine, and Exparel. Hand (N Y) 2016;11(2):177–83.

Foot and Ankle

Multimodal Analgesia in Foot and Ankle Surgery

Jessica M. Kohring, MD[a],*, Nathan G. Orgain, MD[b]

KEYWORDS

- Multimodal • Analgesia • Foot and ankle • Surgery • Orthopedics

---

KEY POINTS

- Recent advances in multimodal analgesia have allowed most foot and ankle surgery to be performed in ambulatory outpatient surgical centers.
- Multimodal analgesia focuses on improving postoperative pain while limiting adverse effects of individual agents, which allows less reliance on opioid pain medications and a decrease in their adverse effects.
- Numerous oral pain medications have been used in multimodal therapy, including nonsteroidal anti-inflammatory drugs (NSAIDs) and selective cyclooxygenase-2 (COX-2) inhibitors, acetaminophen or paracetamol, neuromodulatory medications (gabapentin and pregabalin), opioid agonists, glucocorticoids, and N-Methyl D-Aspartate (NMDA) antagonists.
- Local anesthesia techniques, including wound infiltration and intra-articular injections, provide excellent pain relief with very few adverse events.
- The combination of local anesthetic techniques or peripheral nerve blocks with supplementation using oral agents should be first-line analgesic therapy for patients undergoing outpatient foot and ankle procedures.

OVERVIEW

There has been a growing interest in alternative therapies for pain management following orthopedic procedures. In the past, opioid pain medications have been relied on as the treatment of choice for postoperative pain control. Recent progress in surgical and acute pain management strategies have allowed for most patients undergoing foot and ankle surgery to be performed on in ambulatory outpatient surgical centers. This article reviews multimodal analgesia options in the setting of perioperative foot and ankle surgery.

There are more than 90 million orthopedic procedures performed each year in the United States.[1] Of these procedures, 35 million are performed in ambulatory centers.[2] Orthopedic patients report the highest incidence of pain compared with other types of surgical procedures, with greater than 50% of patients having suboptimal pain control.[3] Postoperative pain is the most important concern among patients and is the most common reason for fear and avoidance of surgery.[4]

PERIOPERATIVE SURGICAL HOME

Pain management is a multifaceted system involving patients, physicians, hospitals, and health care organizations. The concept of a perioperative surgical home involves collaboration between the patient, the orthopedic surgeon, the anesthesiologist, and primary care or

---

Disclosure Statement: The authors did not receive grants or outside funding in support of their research for or preparation of this article. They did not receive payments or other benefits, or a commitment or agreement to provide such benefits from a commercial entity.

[a] Department of Orthopaedics, The University of Utah, 590 Wakara Way, Salt Lake City, UT 84108, USA;
[b] Department of Anesthesiology, The University of Utah, SOM 3C444, 30 North 1900 East, Salt Lake City, UT 84132, USA
* Corresponding author.
E-mail address: jessica.kohring@hsc.utah.edu

internal medicine provider. The perioperative surgical home provides a continuum of patient-focused perioperative care in the preoperative, intraoperative, and postoperative periods to allow for preoperative optimization, safe intraoperative care, and smooth transitions postoperatively through rehabilitation and back to primary care. The goal of this system is to improve outcomes following orthopedic surgery. Communication among these team members is essential to produce good perioperative outcomes and transitions after surgery. There are increased complications associated with increased postoperative pain.[5] Prolonged hospitalization, increased readmission rate, higher costs, and slower recovery are associated with poorer postoperative pain control.[3,6,7] Management of patient expectations for the preoperative, perioperative, and postoperative course in regard to rehabilitation and pain are key in improving outcomes following surgery. Multimodal analgesia is an important component in this pain management system.

OPIOID EPIDEMIC

Traditionally, opioid analgesics have been the cornerstone of postoperative analgesia following orthopedic surgery. Opioids as the sole source of analgesia are associated with significant side effects, and opioid-related adverse events occur more frequently with increased age, obesity, chronic obstructive pulmonary disease, obstructive sleep apnea, and hepatic and renal impairment.[8] A retrospective review of a large national hospital database of 319,898 surgeries showed a 12.2% rate of opioid-related adverse events. Patients who experienced opioid-related adverse events had a higher adjusted mean cost of hospitalization, a greater length of stay, and were more likely to be readmitted.[6] Hospitalizations and emergency department visits due to opioid abuse and misuse continue to increase. Between 2002 and 2012, hospitalization rates for opioid overuse among adults 18 years or older increased by greater than 60%.[9] From 2006 to 2010, emergency department visits involving nonmedical use of opioids increased by 112%. Since 2003, opioid analgesics have been the cause of more deaths from overdose than cocaine and heroine combined.[10] The increase in abuse, accidental death, and the high health care costs associated with opioid abuse has put an emphasis on alternative methods for perioperative pain control, as well as legislation aimed at restricting opioid prescriptions.

MULTIMODAL ANALGESIA

Recent gains in the area of multimodal analgesia have led to effective alternative methods of pain control. Multimodal analgesia focuses on improving postoperative pain while limiting adverse effects of individual agents. Combining pharmacologic and other modalities addresses multiple pain mechanisms while reducing adverse effects through the use of lower doses of individual modalities.[11] Multimodal therapy can shorten hospital stays, minimize use of narcotics, decrease pain scores, reduce opioid adverse effects, decrease times to reach rehabilitation milestones, and improve patient outcomes.[12,13] Effective pain control requires combined drug synergy effects that block generation and perception of pain at several different stages in the pain pathway.[14] Neuraxial and regional anesthesia block transmission of noxious stimuli in sensory neurons before it starts, and multimodal analgesia potentiates the effect of concomitant medications.[13] The simultaneous use of 2 or more analgesics that act at different sites and receptor pathways within the central and peripheral nervous systems work to reduce pain and minimize opioid use (Fig. 1).[14,15] Various oral medications have been used in multimodal therapy, including nonsteroidal anti-inflammatory drugs (NSAIDs) and cyclooxygenase (COX)-2 inhibitors, acetaminophen or paracetamol, neuromodulatory medications (gabapentin and pregabalin), opioid agonists, steroids, and N-methyl D-aspartate (NMDA) antagonists.

There is limited literature in foot and ankle surgery regarding the use of multimodal pain regimens. A multimodal pain protocol suggested by Michelson and colleagues[16] seems to have favorable outcomes in patients undergoing ankle and hindfoot fusions. This multimodal pain protocol consisted of preoperative oral administration of extended-release oxycodone (10 mg), celecoxib (200 mg), pregabalin (75 mg), acetaminophen (1gm), and prednisone (40 mg). The postoperative pain regimen included oral extended-release oxycodone (10 mg every 12 hours), celecoxib (200 mg every 12 hours), and acetaminophen (1000 mg every 6 hours). Short-acting oxycodone (5–20 mg every 4 hours) was provided for breakthrough pain. Subjects were then discharged with prescriptions for 2 days of long-acting oxycodone, 2 weeks of celecoxib, and 2 weeks of short-acting oxycodone. The traditional protocol included no preoperative medications and the use of a patient-controlled analgesia–delivered

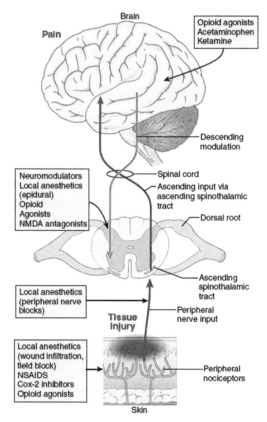

Fig. 1. The pain pathway in the central and peripheral nervous systems and the sites of action for each class of medication. COX-2, cyclooxygenase-2; NMDA, N-methyl D-aspartate; NSAIDs, nonsteroidal anti-inflammatory drugs.

parenteral opioid (dilaudid or morphine). The choice of the pain control protocol was based on surgeon preference. In this retrospective review, 175 subjects received the multimodal postoperative analgesia protocol, and 45 subjects received the traditional pain management. The multimodal protocol subjects had significantly shorter length of hospital stays, controlling for complexity of the surgery performed. Multimodal analgesia works to limit the adverse effects of opioids, improve postoperative pain, and decrease length of hospital stay.

COMPONENTS OF MULTIMODAL ANALGESIA
Nonsteroidal Anti-inflammatory Drugs
NSAIDs are commonly used medications to treat pain and inflammation (Table 1). The mechanism of action for this class of drugs is to inhibit the enzyme COX, which blocks the production of prostaglandins. Two isoenzymes of cyclooxygenase have been identified: COX-1 and COX-2.

The COX-2 isoenzyme is involved primarily in the production of prostaglandins that lead to the inflammatory response and pain perception.[17] The COX-1 isoenzyme has multiple physiologic roles, including platelet, kidney, and gastrointestinal tract functions. Nonspecific NSAIDs are effective for relieving pain and inflammation with the inhibition of the COX-2 isoenzyme, but they are also associated with platelet dysfunction, gastrointestinal and renal toxicity, increasing cardiovascular event risk, and the potential for impaired bone and tendon healing.[17]

Two randomized, controlled trials looking at the use of postoperative diclofenac (nonselective COX) versus placebo in subjects who underwent foot and ankle surgery found that the diclofenac groups in both studies had significantly decreased postoperative pain for 5 days after surgery.[18,19] The medications were well tolerated in both studies with high subject satisfaction and decreased need for supplemental narcotic analgesia compared with the placebo group.[18,19]

The COX-2-specific NSAIDs, referred to as coxibs, have been developed to reduce or eliminate many unwanted side effects of nonselective NSAIDs, specifically the gastrointestinal and platelet effects. Previous coxibs, including rofecoxib and valdecoxib, have been removed from the market due to concerns that they are associated with increased cardiovascular risk.[20] Selective COX-2 inhibitors have been found to be quite effective in postoperative pain control in patients undergoing orthopedic procedures. Brattwall and colleagues[21] conducted a trial comparing postoperative etoricoxib versus tramadol in subjects undergoing bunion surgery. The etoricoxib group had significantly decreased pain scores, increased satisfaction, and decreased side effects compared with the tramadol group.

The use of NSAIDs and selective COX-2 inhibitors in orthopedic surgery remains controversial. There have been numerous studies suggesting the inhibitory effects of NSAIDs on bone healing in animal models, but no definitive research to date has shown evidence of an actual effect in humans.[22–27] More recent literature has started to examine if NSAIDs and coxibs have an impact on soft tissue healing.[25,28,29] A recent systematic review found that short-term, low-dose use of NSAIDs and COX-2 inhibitors do not seem to have detrimental effects on soft tissue healing but may show an inhibitory effect in bony healing. Based on the available literature, the investigators recommended the use of NSAIDs and coxibs for soft tissue procedures,

Table 1
Multimodal analgesia medication classes

Drug Category	Mechanism of Action	Dosing	Advantages	Disadvantages
NSAIDs				
Ibuprofen (PO)	COX inhibitor (nonspecific)	400–800 mg q 6 h	No addictive potential, OTC, efficacious analgesic	Potential renal toxicity, platelet inhibition, inhibition of bone & soft tissue healing, gastric mucosa effects
Ketorolac (IV)		15–30 mg q 6 h (limit to 6 doses total)	Potent analgesic	Cardiovascular risk, gastric mucosa effects, higher gastric mucosa toxicity compared with other NSAIDs
Celexicob	COX-2 inhibitor (specific)	200 mg q 12 h	Reduced platelet effect, reduced gastric toxicity	Increased cardiovascular risk, potential renal toxicity
Acetaminophen	CNS inhibition of COX, modulation of central serotonin		Well tolerated	Caution with hepatic disease
Acetaminophen (PO)		Up to 1 g q 6 h	Inexpensive	May not produce therapeutic levels in perioperative period
Paracetamol (IV)		Up to 1 g q 6 h	Reliable CNS levels in perioperative period	Expensive
Neuromodulatory Medications	Voltage-dependent calcium channels in CNS or PNS		Reduces opioid use & opioid-related side effects	
Gabapentin (PO)		300 mg tid		Dizziness, drowsiness, ataxia, fatigue
Pregabalin (PO)		75–100 mg q 12 h		Dizziness, somnolence, visual disturbances
Opioid Agonist				Constipation, nausea, pruiritis, respiratory depression
Oxycodone (PO)	Mu receptor agonist	5–15 mg q 3-6 h		
Combined Opioid Agonist or Norepinephrine-SSRIs	Mu agonist or inhibitor of norepine phrine-serotonin reuptake			Caution use with other SSRIs such as SSRI antidepressants

Drug Category	Mechanism of Action	Dosing	Advantages	Disadvantages
Tramadol (PO)	Serotonin & norepinephrine uptake inhibitor	50–100 mg q 6 h	Lower risk of tolerance, dependence	Flushing, dizziness, headache, drowsiness, insomnia
Tapentadol (PO)	Norepinephrine reuptake inhibitor only	50–75 mg q 6 h	Lower risk of tolerance, dependence, nausea, constipation	Dizziness, drowsiness, fatigue, insomnia
Glucocorticoids				
Dexamethasone (PO)		0.1 mg/kg dose preoperative or postoperative	Decrease nausea, decrease opioid use	Cardiovascular risk, CNS effects, decreased glucose tolerance
NMDA Antagonist	Modulate central sensitization of nociceptive stimulation			
Ketamine (IV)		0.5 mg/kg initial bolus, 0.1 mg/kg/h infusion intraoperative, can continue same dose postoperative for 48 h	Less opioid requirements postoperative	Agitation, confusion, hallucinations, muscle tremors, HTN, high abuse potential
Memantine (PO)		Start at 5–10 mg bid, titrate up weekly to 30 mg/d	Well tolerated	Psychosis

Medications in each of these categories can be used concurrently for multimodal analgesia.

Abbreviations: bid, 2 times per day; CNS, central nervous system; IV, intravenous; OTC, over-the-counter; PO, by mouth; q, every; qid, 4 times per day; SSRI, serotonin reuptake inhibitor; tid, 3 times per day.

but recommended against their use in procedures requiring bone healing.[30]

Acetaminophen and Paracetamol

Oral acetaminophen and paracetamol, its parenteral form, are well-tolerated agents with relatively few side effects that are commonly used in conjunction with opioids for postoperative pain control. The mechanism of action for these agents is not well understood, but they have been shown to inhibit COX in the central nervous system (CNS) and have an effect on central modulation of the serotonin system.[31,32] There seems to be little difference in analgesia effects between the oral and parenteral forms of acetaminophen when therapeutic levels are maintained. A randomized, controlled trial of 30 subjects undergoing knee arthroscopy showed that all subjects who received parenteral acetaminophen reached plasma levels in the therapeutic analgesic range. In comparison, less than half of the subjects who received the oral form of the medication received therapeutic analgesic plasma levels. The subjects who received intravenous paracetamol showed a trend toward decreased need for rescue analgesia and a shorter stay in the recovery room.[33]

Neuromodulatory Medications (Gabapentin, Pregabalin)

Gabapentin and pregabalin are gamma-aminobutyric acid analogues that bind to voltage-gated calcium channels in the central and peripheral nervous system and alter the release of excitatory neurotransmitters.[34] Pregabalin has a faster onset, more predictable plasma concentrations, and fewer side effects compared with gabapentin. Peak plasma concentrations are reached within an hour for pregabalin due to its absorption kinetics in the gut versus 3 to 4 hours for gabapentin, which is absorbed by a saturable receptor-mediated route.[34,35] As a result, gabapentin has less reliable bioavailability than pregabalin. Pregabalin is more expensive than gabapentin, but for a brief course in the perioperative period it can often be covered.[34] The most common side effects associated with pregabalin are dizziness, visual disturbances, and somnolence. As an adjunct for pain control, the typical starting dose is 75 mg 2 times per day, although effective doses for reducing perioperative opioid requirements range up to 150 mg 2 times per day.[34] Pregabalin has been found to reduce opioid requirements and opioid-related side effects in multiple perioperative settings and procedures.[35,36] Subjects treated with pregabalin in the perioperative period have shown a lower incidence of chronic pain associated with surgery.[37,38] A randomized, placebo-controlled, double-blind study of 240 subjects undergoing total knee arthroplasty found that the 120 subjects who received perioperative pregabalin showed significantly lower rates of neuropathic pain, less opioid consumption, and improved functional rehabilitation compared with the placebo group at 6 months after surgery.[36]

Opioid Agonists (Tramadol and Tapentadol)

Opioid medications work through agonistic activity at the mu opioid receptor within the CNS. Opioids remain the mainstay analgesic prescribed by most clinicians despite their addictive potential and side-effect profile. The most common opioid-related side effects include nausea, constipation, pruritus, and ventilatory depression. All opioid medications seem to have similar side-effect profiles and analgesic effects when compared in equivalent doses.[39,40] Multimodal analgesia allows for a reduction in opioid dose requirements and thus opioid-related side effects.[41] In subjects undergoing corrective bunion surgery, Richards and colleagues[42] found that those subjects randomized to receive a combination of oral immediate-release morphine and oxycodone had significantly decreased pain and side effects compared with subjects who received higher doses of individual oral doses of morphine or oxycodone.

Tramadol and tapentdaol are medications with a mechanism of action at both the opioid receptor and via monoamine reuptake inhibition.[43,44] Tramadol inhibits the reuptake of both serotonin and norepinephrine; tapentadol only affects norepinephrine levels.[45] These medications do not rely on mu opioid agonist activity as their sole mechanism for analgesia. There is evidence to suggest that these analgesics may be associated with less respiratory depression than conventional opioids at similar levels of dosing.[46–49] Tapentadol has a lower incidence of gastrointestinal side effects, including nausea, vomiting, and constipation, compared with other commonly prescribed opioids.[50] Tramadol has not been associated with the same decrease in gastrointestinal side effects as tapentadol. Care must be taken in prescribing these medications with drugs whose mechanism of action also involve increasing CNS serotonin and norepinephrine levels,[44] such as commonly prescribed serotonin reuptake inhibitors and selective norepinephrine reuptake inhibitors. Serotonin syndrome is a potentially life-threatening condition that may develop in patients with increased CNS serotonin or norepinephrine concentrations. Agitation, delirium, and autonomic dysfunction, including diaphoresis, tachycardia, hyperthermia, as well as neuromuscular hyperactivity manifesting as muscle rigidity and myoclonus, are the main clinical findings in patients presenting with serotonin syndrome.[44]

Stegmann and colleagues[51] conducted a randomized, double-blind, controlled trial of immediate-release tapentadol versus immediate-release oxycodone versus placebo in subjects undergoing a first metatarsal osteotomy. The subjects randomized to the tapentadol and oxycodone groups had significantly less pain postoperatively compared with the placebo group at comparable rates. The subjects taking tapentadol had lower rates of nausea, dizziness, vomiting, and constipation compared with the subjects taking oxycodone. There is evidence to suggest that tapentadol shows comparable analgesia to oxycodone with fewer side effects in patients undergoing foot surgery.

Glucocorticoids

Glucocorticoid administration, in the perioperative period, is reported to reduce pain, shorten hospital stay, and decrease time back to work following both inpatient and outpatient orthopedic surgeries.[52,53] Single-dose preoperative or 24-hour perioperative use of high-dose glucocorticoids has been shown to be safe without evidence of increased risk for postoperative wound infections or other complications.[54,55] Preoperative administration of intramuscular betamethasone improved pain relief during the first 24 hours postoperatively in a study of orthopedic day-surgery subjects.[52] A randomized, controlled trial of 50 subjects undergoing first metatarsal osteotomy, as a day-surgery procedure, were randomized to receive either 9 mg oral dexamethasone or placebo preoperatively and 24 hours postoperatively. The investigators found significantly lower pain scores, less nausea, and significantly less oxycodone consumption in the dexamethasone group in the acute postoperative period.[56]

N-Methyl D-Aspartate Antagonists (Ketamine and Memantine)

Ketamine is an NMDA antagonist with analgesic properties that modulate central sensitization of nociceptive stimulation. NMDA receptors are involved in the perception of postoperative pain due to their role in neuronal plasticity leading to central sensitization.[57] Ketamine is administered intravenously with an initial bolus of 0.5 mg/kg, followed by continuous infusion of 3 µg/kg/min during surgery, and 1.5 µg/kg/min for the following 48 hours.[58] When used in combination with peripheral nerve blocks, several trials have shown that subjects undergoing total knee arthroplasty and knee arthroscopy require significantly less morphine than the control groups who only received peripheral nerve blocks.[59,60] Ketamine is associated with agitation, confusion, hallucinations, muscle tremors, hypertension, and thus its use should be monitored closely.[58] Memantine is an orally available noncompetitive NMDA receptor antagonist used to treat moderate to severe Alzheimer dementia.[61] It has also been found to be an effective analgesic and may prove to be more useful than ketamine as an analgesia adjunct in decreasing the risk for the development of postoperative chronic pain.[61]

Combination Therapies

Combination therapies of acetaminophen (or paracetamol) and NSAIDs are effective analgesia options in subjects undergoing orthopedic procedures. A systematic review of the literature, including 21 studies, showed that the combination of paracetamol and an NSAID, including ibuprofen, diclofenac, aspirin, tenoxicam, rofecoxib, ketoprofen, and ketorolac, had improved analgesia as compared with either medication alone in surgical subjects.[62]

Although limited in data, the combination of gabapentin plus celexicob on postoperative pain after orthopedic procedures has been found to be an effective treatment therapy. A randomized, double-blind, controlled trial of 114 subjects who underwent elective laminectomy were assigned to gabapentin alone (900 mg daily), gabapentin (300 mg 2 times per day) plus celexicob (200 mg 2 times per day), or placebo. Subjects who received the combination therapy gabapentin plus celexicob had significantly lower mean pain severity scores and morphine consumption for 24 hours postoperatively than the gabapentin alone or the placebo groups. These subjects also had significantly higher postoperative satisfaction. The gabapentin-only group experienced significantly more drowsiness than the other 2 groups.[63]

Intra-articular Injections

Intra-articular injection of local anesthetics is commonly used for pain relief after arthroscopy in orthopedic procedures. The use of a 1-time intra-articular injection of bupivacaine, morphine, and methylprednisolone after ankle arthroscopy has been shown to decrease postoperative pain and reduction in impairment.[64] Intra-articular injections of bupivacaine following knee and ankle arthroscopic procedures have been shown to be safe and effective in decreasing postoperative pain scores and additional analgesic requirements.[65-68]

Local Wound Infiltration

Local wound infiltration with local anesthetic or a multidrug injection is a convenient, safe, and effective option for pain control. It has been widely used after total knee and hip arthroplasties. It seems to have favorable outcomes in the foot and ankle literature, as well as in the few studies looking at the effect of local wound infiltration on postoperative pain and outcomes. Kim and colleagues[69] injected ropivacaine, morphine, ketorolac, and epinephrine in the wounds of subjects undergoing bilateral hallux valgus correction surgery. The contralateral side was injected with normal saline. Subjects reported significantly less pain on the local injection side compared with the contralateral side. Similar results were found in a study of subjects undergoing ankle supramalleolar osteotomies. Thirty-one subjects were randomized to receive a local wound injection of ropivacaine, morphine, ketorolac, and epinephrine before wound closure. Subjects receiving this injection reported significantly less postoperative pain and had decreased opioid requirements compared with the placebo group.[69]

Liposomal bupivacaine is a local anesthetic that allows for extended, sustained release of bupivacaine over 72 hours without reaching systemically toxic levels.[70,71] It is approved by the US Food and Drug Administration for single-dose infiltration into the surgical site to produce postsurgical analgesia. In a case-control study by Robbins and colleagues,[72] local liposomal bupivacaine was injected into the wounds of 20 subjects undergoing forefoot surgery at the time of closure. These subjects showed a trend toward lower postoperative pain scores and fewer pain medication refills compared with the control group. Both groups received a standard multimodal analgesic regimen, including celocoxib, preoperatively and postoperatively, and oral narcotics. Additionally, there was no significant difference between the groups for wound infection. Golf and colleagues[73] conducted a randomized, placebo-controlled trial of liposomal bupivacaine versus placebo in 193 subjects undergoing bunion surgery. Before closure, wound infiltration of liposomal bupivacaine was administered. The 97 subjects treated with liposomal bupivacaine had significantly less pain than the control group postoperatively. In addition, more subjects in the extended-release bupivacaine group avoided the use of opioid rescue medication during the first 24 hours and were pain-free up to 48 hours after surgery. Liposomal bupivacaine has been shown to be an effective adjunct to multimodal postoperative pain regimens in many other orthopedic procedures. In addition, it has been associated with decreased postoperative narcotic requirements,[28,73,74] shorter inpatient length of stay,[28,75] and lower inpatient costs.[28,75] No studies have shown an effect on wound healing[28,73-76] or union when compared with plain bupivacaine or a placebo.[73]

SUMMARY

The use of multimodal analgesia in foot and ankle surgery provides superior pain relief, reduction in dependence on opioids, and decreased opioid-related side effects. Most of the available literature in foot and ankle surgery used dual-modality analgesia with 1 drug versus a placebo and the use of opioids as rescue medications. The combination of acetaminophen or paracetamol and NSAIDs and/or COX-2 inhibitors has been shown to provide improved pain relief compared with either drug alone. Local anesthesia techniques, including wound infiltration and intra-articular injections, provide excellent pain relief with very few adverse events. These modalities should be considered for first-line analgesic therapy with supplementation using oral agents for day-surgery patients. The synergistic effects of multiple medications provide effective analgesia, reduce opioid use and side effects, quicken mobilization and recovery, decrease length of hospital stays, reduce rates of readmission, and improve patient satisfaction scores. Multimodal pain management will continue to evolve with the goal to minimize opioid use and improve postoperative patient outcomes.[3,6,7,77]

EXAMPLE CASE

Here is a case example of a sample regimen for multimodal analgesia used for an outpatient foot and ankle patient:

> Patient: A 61-year-old man presenting for a medializing calcaneal osteotomy with a posterior tibial tendon and spring ligament repair (weight 88 kg).
> Past medical history: hypertension, type II diabetes, knee osteoarthritis.
> Current medications: lisinopril, metformin (held day of surgery), ibuprofen as needed for arthritis (none taken day of surgery). The patient does not consume any opioids.
> Laboratory tests: normal creatinine and fasting glucose.

Multimodal preoperative combinations

1. Acetaminophen 650 to 975 mg orally
2. Celexicob 200 to 400 mg orally
3. Pregabalin 75 to 150 mg orally (could substitute gabapentin 300 mg orally)
4. Tapentadol 50 to 100 mg orally (could substitute oxycodone 5–10 mg orally if opioid-naïve due to cost)
5. Consideration of regional anesthesia nerve blocks appropriate to surgery, for example, sciatic or popliteal fossa nerve block or catheter with or without saphenous nerve or adductor canal block.

The multimodal postoperative regimen duration of treatment is determined based on the patient, surgical, and anticipated recovery factors. The as-needed medications can be applied in a step-wise manner as the patient's pain control requirements necessitates:

1. Acetaminophen 650 mg orally every 6 hours scheduled
2. Pregabalin 75 mg orally every 12 hours scheduled (7–10 days as indicated by surgical procedure)
3. Celecoxib 200 mg orally every 12 hours as needed (short course 3–7 days, can

substitute other NSAID for procedures with low risk of nonunion; do not recommend use of any type of NSAID for patients with a high risk of nonunion after surgery)
4. Either:
    a. Tapentadol 50 mg orally every 12 hours as needed (can titrate up to 100 mg every 12 hours as needed)
    b. Oxycodone 5 to 15 mg orally every 12 hours as needed.

In regard to multimodal pain regimens, clinical judgment must always be applied to adjust, omit, or substitute appropriate medications, doses, intervals, and durations to ensure safe and optimal care.

REFERENCES

1. DeFrances CJ, Lucas CA, Buie VC, et al. 2006 National Hospital Discharge Survey. Natl Health Stat Report 2008;30(5):1–20.
2. Cullen KA, Hall MJ, Golosinskiy A. Ambulatory surgery in the United States, 2006. Natl Health Stat Report 2009;(11):1–25.
3. Apfelbaum JL, Chen C, Mehta SS, et al. Postoperative pain experience: results from a national survey suggest postoperative pain continues to be undermanaged. Anesth Analg 2003;97(2):534–40. table of contents.
4. Mannion AF, Kampfen S, Munzinger U, et al. The role of patient expectations in predicting outcome after total knee arthroplasty. Arthritis Res Ther 2009;11(5):R139.
5. Wu CL, Raja SN. Treatment of acute postoperative pain. Lancet 2011;377(9784):2215–25.
6. Oderda GM, Gan TJ, Johnson BH, et al. Effect of opioid-related adverse events on outcomes in selected surgical patients. J Pain Palliat Care Pharmacother 2013;27(1):62–70.
7. Popping DM, Zahn PK, Van Aken HK, et al. Effectiveness and safety of postoperative pain management: a survey of 18 925 consecutive patients between 1998 and 2006 (2nd revision): a database analysis of prospectively raised data. Br J Anaesth 2008;101(6):832–40.
8. Barrington JW, Halaszynski TM, Sinatra RS, Expert Working Group On Anesthesia And Orthopaedics Critical Issues In Hip And Knee Replacement Arthroplasty FT. Perioperative pain management in hip and knee replacement surgery. Am J Orthop (Belle Mead NJ) 2014;43(4 Suppl):S1–16.
9. Owens PL, Barrett ML, Weiss AJ, et al. Hospital Inpatient Utilization Related to Opioid Overuse Among Adults, 1993-2012: Statistical Brief #177. Healthcare Cost and Utilization Project (HCUP) Statistical Briefs. Rockville (MD): 2006.
10. Centers for Disease Control and Prevention. CDC grand rounds: prescription drug overdoses - a U.S. epidemic. MMWR Morb Mortal Wkly Rep 2012;61(1):10–3.
11. Nett MP. Postoperative pain management. Orthopedics 2010;33(9 Suppl):23–6.
12. Ekman EF, Koman LA. Acute pain following musculoskeletal injuries and orthopaedic surgery: mechanisms and management. Instr Course Lect 2005;54:21–33.
13. Kehlet H, Wilmore DW. Multimodal strategies to improve surgical outcome. Am J Surg 2002;183(6):630–41.
14. Kehlet H, Dahl JB. The value of "multimodal" or "balanced analgesia" in postoperative pain treatment. Anesth Analg 1993;77(5):1048–56.
15. Buvanendran A, Kroin JS. Multimodal analgesia for controlling acute postoperative pain. Curr Opin Anaesthesiol 2009;22(5):588–93.
16. Michelson JD, Addante RA, Charlson MD. Multimodal analgesia therapy reduces length of hospitalization in patients undergoing fusions of the ankle and hindfoot. Foot Ankle Int 2013;34(11):1526–34.
17. Botting RM. Mechanism of action of acetaminophen: is there a cyclooxygenase 3? Clin Infect Dis 2000;31(Suppl 5):S202–10.
18. Riff DS, Duckor S, Gottlieb I, et al. Diclofenac potassium liquid-filled soft gelatin capsules in the management of patients with postbunionectomy pain: a Phase III, multicenter, randomized, double-blind, placebo-controlled study conducted over 5 days. Clin Ther 2009;31(10):2072–85.
19. Daniels SE, Baum DR, Clark F, et al. Diclofenac potassium liquid-filled soft gelatin capsules for the treatment of postbunionectomy pain. Curr Med Res Opin 2010;26(10):2375–84.
20. Hinz B, Renner B, Brune K. Drug insight: cyclooxygenase-2 inhibitors–a critical appraisal. Nat Clin Pract Rheumatol 2007;3(10):552–60 [quiz: 551]. p following 589.
21. Brattwall M, Turan I, Jakobsson J. Pain management after elective hallux valgus surgery: a prospective randomized double-blind study comparing etoricoxib and tramadol. Anesth Analg 2010;111(2):544–9.
22. Allen HL, Wase A, Bear WT. Indomethacin and aspirin: effect of nonsteroidal anti-inflammatory agents on the rate of fracture repair in the rat. Acta Orthop Scand 1980;51(4):595–600.
23. Beck A, Krischak G, Sorg T, et al. Influence of diclofenac (group of nonsteroidal anti-inflammatory drugs) on fracture healing. Arch Orthop Trauma Surg 2003;123(7):327–32.
24. Brown KM, Saunders MM, Kirsch T, et al. Effect of COX-2-specific inhibition on fracture-healing in the rat femur. J Bone Joint Surg Am 2004;86A(1):116–23.

25. Dimmen S, Engebretsen L, Nordsletten L, et al. Negative effects of parecoxib and indomethacin on tendon healing: an experimental study in rats. Knee Surg Sports Traumatol Arthrosc 2009;17(7): 835–9.

26. Dimmen S, Nordsletten L, Madsen JE. Parecoxib and indomethacin delay early fracture healing: a study in rats. Clin Orthop Relat Res 2009;467(8): 1992–9.

27. Simon AM, O'Connor JP. Dose and time-dependent effects of cyclooxygenase-2 inhibition on fracture-healing. J Bone Joint Surg Am 2007; 89(3):500–11.

28. Cohen SM. Extended pain relief trial utilizing infiltration of Exparel((R)), a long-acting multivesicular liposome formulation of bupivacaine: a Phase IV health economic trial in adult patients undergoing open colectomy. J Pain Res 2012;5: 567–72.

29. Dahners LE, Gilbert JA, Lester GE, et al. The effect of a nonsteroidal antiinflammatory drug on the healing of ligaments. Am J Sports Med 1988; 16(6):641–6.

30. Chen MR, Dragoo JL. The effect of nonsteroidal anti-inflammatory drugs on tissue healing. Knee Surg Sports Traumatol Arthrosc 2013;21(3):540–9.

31. Graham GG, Scott KF. Mechanism of action of paracetamol. Am J Ther 2005;12(1):46–55.

32. Graham GG, Scott KF, Day RO. Tolerability of paracetamol. Drug Saf 2005;28(3):227–40.

33. Brett CN, Barnett SG, Pearson J. Postoperative plasma paracetamol levels following oral or intravenous paracetamol administration: a double-blind randomised controlled trial. Anaesth Intensive Care 2012;40(1):166–71.

34. Bockbrader HN, Radulovic LL, Posvar EL, et al. Clinical pharmacokinetics of pregabalin in healthy volunteers. J Clin Pharmacol 2010;50(8):941–50.

35. Gajraj NM. Pregabalin: its pharmacology and use in pain management. Anesth Analg 2007;105(6): 1805–15.

36. Buvanendran A, Kroin JS, Della Valle CJ, et al. Perioperative oral pregabalin reduces chronic pain after total knee arthroplasty: a prospective, randomized, controlled trial. Anesth Analg 2010; 110(1):199–207.

37. Kim JC, Choi YS, Kim KN, et al. Effective dose of peri-operative oral pregabalin as an adjunct to multimodal analgesic regimen in lumbar spinal fusion surgery. Spine (Phila Pa 1976) 2011;36(6): 428–33.

38. Zhang J, Ho KY, Wang Y. Efficacy of pregabalin in acute postoperative pain: a meta-analysis. Br J Anaesth 2011;106(4):454–62.

39. Benyamin R, Trescot AM, Datta S, et al. Opioid complications and side effects. Pain Physician 2008;11(2 Suppl):S105–20.

40. Swegle JM, Logemann C. Management of common opioid-induced adverse effects. Am Fam Physician 2006;74(8):1347–54.

41. Maheshwari AV, Blum YC, Shekhar L, et al. Multimodal pain management after total hip and knee arthroplasty at the Ranawat Orthopaedic Center. Clin Orthop Relat Res 2009;467(6):1418–23.

42. Richards P, Riff D, Kelen R, et al. Analgesic and adverse effects of a fixed-ratio morphine-oxycodone combination (MoxDuo) in the treatment of postoperative pain. J Opioid Manag 2011;7(3): 217–28.

43. Dayer P, Desmeules J, Collart L. Pharmacology of tramadol. Drugs 1997;53(Suppl 2):18–24 [in French].

44. Nossaman VE, Ramadhyani U, Kadowitz PJ, et al. Advances in perioperative pain management: use of medications with dual analgesic mechanisms, tramadol & tapentadol. Anesthesiol Clin 2010; 28(4):647–66.

45. Frampton JE. Tapentadol immediate release: a review of its use in the treatment of moderate to severe acute pain. Drugs 2010;70(13):1719–43.

46. Houmes RJ, Voets MA, Verkaaik A, et al. Efficacy and safety of tramadol versus morphine for moderate and severe postoperative pain with special regard to respiratory depression. Anesth Analg 1992;74(4):510–4.

47. Prommer EE. Tramadol: does it have a role in cancer pain management? J Opioid Manag 2005;1(3): 131–8.

48. Radbruch L, Grond S, Lehmann KA. A risk-benefit assessment of tramadol in the management of pain. Drug Saf 1996;15(1):8–29.

49. Shipton EA. Tramadol–present and future. Anaesth Intensive Care 2000;28(4):363–74.

50. Hartrick CT. Tapentadol immediate release for the relief of moderate-to-severe acute pain. Expert Opin Pharmacother 2009;10(16):2687–96.

51. Stegmann JU, Weber H, Steup A, et al. The efficacy and tolerability of multiple-dose tapentadol immediate release for the relief of acute pain following orthopedic (bunionectomy) surgery. Curr Med Res Opin 2008;24(11):3185–96.

52. Aasboe V, Raeder JC, Groegaard B. Betamethasone reduces postoperative pain and nausea after ambulatory surgery. Anesth Analg 1998;87(2): 319–23.

53. Lundin A, Magnuson A, Axelsson K, et al. The effect of perioperative corticosteroids on the outcome of microscopic lumbar disc surgery. Eur Spine J 2003; 12(6):625–30.

54. Henzi I, Walder B, Tramer MR. Dexamethasone for the prevention of postoperative nausea and vomiting: a quantitative systematic review. Anesth Analg 2000;90(1):186–94.

55. Sauerland S, Nagelschmidt M, Mallmann P, et al. Risks and benefits of preoperative high dose

methylprednisolone in surgical patients: a systematic review. Drug Saf 2000;23(5):449–61.

56. Mattila K, Kontinen VK, Kalso E, et al. Dexamethasone decreases oxycodone consumption following osteotomy of the first metatarsal bone: a randomized controlled trial in day surgery. Acta Anaesthesiol Scand 2010;54(3):268–76.

57. Sunder RA, Toshniwal G, Dureja GP. Ketamine as an adjuvant in sympathetic blocks for management of central sensitization following peripheral nerve injury. J Brachial Plex Peripher Nerve Inj 2008;3:22.

58. Koyyalamudi V, Sen S, Patil S, et al. Adjuvant agents in regional anesthesia in the ambulatory setting. Curr Pain Headache Rep 2017;21(1):6.

59. Adam F, Chauvin M, Du Manoir B, et al. Small-dose ketamine infusion improves postoperative analgesia and rehabilitation after total knee arthroplasty. Anesth Analg 2005;100(2):475–80.

60. Menigaux C, Guignard B, Fletcher D, et al. Intraoperative small-dose ketamine enhances analgesia after outpatient knee arthroscopy. Anesth Analg 2001;93(3):606–12.

61. Young A, Buvanendran A. Recent advances in multimodal analgesia. Anesthesiol Clin 2012;30(1):91–100.

62. Ong CK, Seymour RA, Lirk P, et al. Combining paracetamol (acetaminophen) with nonsteroidal antiinflammatory drugs: a qualitative systematic review of analgesic efficacy for acute postoperative pain. Anesth Analg 2010;110(4):1170–9.

63. Vasigh A, Jaafarpour M, Khajavikhan J, et al. The effect of gabapentin plus celecoxib on pain and associated complications after laminectomy. J Clin Diagn Res 2016;10(3):UC04–8.

64. Rasmussen S, Lorentzen JS, Larsen AS, et al. Combined intra-articular glucocorticoid, bupivacaine and morphine reduces pain and convalescence after diagnostic knee arthroscopy. Acta Orthop Scand 2002;73(2):175–8.

65. Chirwa SS, MacLeod BA, Day B. Intraarticular bupivacaine (Marcaine) after arthroscopic meniscectomy: a randomized double-blind controlled study. Arthroscopy 1989;5(1):33–5.

66. Kaeding CC, Hill JA, Katz J, et al. Bupivacaine use after knee arthroscopy: pharmacokinetics and pain control study. Arthroscopy 1990;6(1):33–9.

67. Katz JA, Kaeding CS, Hill JR, et al. The pharmacokinetics of bupivacaine when injected intra-articularly after knee arthroscopy. Anesth Analg 1988;67(9):872–5.

68. Middleton F, Coakes J, Umarji S, et al. The efficacy of intra-articular bupivacaine for relief of pain following arthroscopy of the ankle. J Bone Joint Surg Br 2006;88(12):1603–5.

69. Kim YS, Kim BS, Koh YG, et al. Efficacy of multimodal drug injection after supramalleolar osteotomy for varus ankle osteoarthritis: a prospective randomized study. J Orthop Sci 2016;21(3):316–22.

70. Naseem A, Harada T, Wang D, et al. Bupivacaine extended release liposome injection does not prolong QTc interval in a thorough QT/QTc study in healthy volunteers. J Clin Pharmacol 2012;52(9):1441–7.

71. Viscusi ER, Sinatra R, Onel E, et al. The safety of liposome bupivacaine, a novel local analgesic formulation. Clin J Pain 2014;30(2):102–10.

72. Robbins J, Green CL, Parekh SG. Liposomal bupivacaine in forefoot surgery. Foot Ankle Int 2015;36(5):503–7.

73. Golf M, Daniels SE, Onel E. A phase 3, randomized, placebo-controlled trial of DepoFoam(R) bupivacaine (extended-release bupivacaine local analgesic) in bunionectomy. Adv Ther 2011;28(9):776–88.

74. Gorfine SR, Onel E, Patou G, et al. Bupivacaine extended-release liposome injection for prolonged postsurgical analgesia in patients undergoing hemorrhoidectomy: a multicenter, randomized, double-blind, placebo-controlled trial. Dis Colon Rectum 2011;54(12):1552–9.

75. Marcet JE, Nfonsam VN, Larach S. An extended pain relief trial utilizing the infiltration of a long-acting Multivesicular liPosome foRmulation of bupiVacaine, EXPAREL (IMPROVE): a Phase IV health economic trial in adult patients undergoing ileostomy reversal. J Pain Res 2013;6:549–55.

76. Bramlett K, Onel E, Viscusi ER, et al. A randomized, double-blind, dose-ranging study comparing wound infiltration of DepoFoam bupivacaine, an extended-release liposomal bupivacaine, to bupivacaine HCl for postsurgical analgesia in total knee arthroplasty. Knee 2012;19(5):530–6.

77. Oderda GM, Said Q, Evans RS, et al. Opioid-related adverse drug events in surgical hospitalizations: impact on costs and length of stay. Ann Pharmacother 2007;41(3):400–6.

Peripheral Nerve Blocks in Foot and Ankle Surgery

Tyler W. Fraser, MD*, Jesse F. Doty, MD

KEYWORDS

- Peripheral nerve block • Foot • Ankle surgery

KEY POINTS

- Increasing outpatient surgery rates necessitates controlling postoperative pain.
- Regional anesthesia decreases hospital length of stay, hospital-associated costs for patients, and perioperative opioid use.
- Postoperative pain has been shown to be factor in patient outcomes.
- Peripheral nerve blocks are a safe alternative to traditional approaches to managing postoperative pain.
- Safe alternative or adjunct to traditional methods for the elderly and those with cardiopulmonary disease.

INTRODUCTION

The advancement of peripheral nerve blocks in foot and ankle surgery has vastly expanded the plethora of choices for pain management in the perioperative period. Without the need for high doses of intravenous pain medication, a larger number of operative procedures can be performed on an outpatient basis, or with shorter observational single-night stays in a hospital setting. These forms of regional anesthesia lead to decreased opioid use and lower reported levels of perioperative pain.[1–4] This may allow patients the option of recovering comfortably at home while incurring lower surgery-related costs.[5] In addition, there are many patients in whom opioids may pose a risk secondary to other medical comorbidities, including those with decreased cognition, dementia, or a previous history of narcotic dependence.

ANATOMY

Sensation to the foot and ankle is provided by the branches of the sciatic nerve and the femoral nerve. Particularly, the femoral nerve terminates as the saphenous nerve, providing sensation to the medial foot. The sciatic nerve divides into the tibial nerve and the common peroneal nerve. The tibial nerve provides plantar foot sensation via the medial and lateral plantar nerves. The common peroneal nerve splits into the superficial peroneal nerve, providing sensation to the dorsal foot, and the deep peroneal nerve, providing sensation to the first web space. The sural nerve is generally derived from branches of both the common peroneal and tibial nerves and provides lateral foot sensation. Targeted anesthesia to the foot and ankle can be delivered to a specific dermatomal distribution by perineural injections of local anesthetic. Alternatively, one can target the sciatic nerve proximally

Disclosure Statement: None (Dr T.W. Fraser). Globus Medical consultant, Arthrex Inc consultant and Speakers Bureau (Dr J.F. Doty).
Department of Orthopaedic Surgery, The University of Tennessee, Erlanger Health System, Chattanooga, TN, USA
* Corresponding author. Department of Orthopaedic Surgery, The University of Tennessee at Chattanooga, 979 East Third Street, Suite 202, Chattanooga, TN 37421.
E-mail address: tyler.fraser4@gmail.com

in the popliteal fossa to target most of the sensation to the foot. A separate injection can then be used medially to block the saphenous nerve and thereby provide anesthesia to the foot (Fig. 1).

Sciatic Nerve
The most commonly used proximal nerve block for foot and ankle surgery is a sciatic nerve block at the level of the popliteal fossa. Generally, the injection is located proximal to the location where the sciatic nerve divides into the tibial nerve and common peroneal nerves. A single injection of anesthetic in this location can provide anesthesia to nearly the entire foot, excluding the medial foot saphenous nerve distribution. In the popliteal fossa, the sciatic nerve lies lateral to the popliteal artery, and is bordered by the heads of the biceps femoris and gastrocnemius on the medial and lateral sides. Success with sciatic nerve blocks has been reported for a wide variety of foot and ankle procedures.[1–3,5–9] Although the sciatic nerve block generally provides adequate anesthesia distally, the common use of thigh tourniquets in foot and ankle surgery may necessitate further anesthesia to avoid thigh discomfort from tourniquet compression. As an alternative, a lower-leg tourniquet around the calf can safely be used and may obviate more proximal anesthesia. Grebing and Coughlin[10] reported the Esmark bandage

provided average tourniquet pressures between 222 and 288 with 3 or 4 wraps, respectively. The complication rate of these ankle level tourniquets was .1%. Michelson and colleagues[11] found no postoperative neurovascular deficits in 454 limbs using cast padding and a standard calf tourniquet (Fig. 2).

Saphenous Nerve
Conventionally, the saphenous nerve was thought to provide sensation to the medial leg and foot. However, there has been much debate about the true contribution to medial foot and ankle sensation, and this is highly variable. Some investigators suggest that the saphenous nerve does not extend past the midfoot, whereas others have found contributions to the first ray, talonavicular, subtalar, and medial ankle joints. These investigators recommend that a saphenous nerve block should be included as a component of the regional block to provide adequate anesthesia during the perioperative period of procedures involving the forefoot.[12–16] At the level of the knee joint, the saphenous nerve can be found between the vastus medialis and sartorius myotendinous junctions. A fascial plane separates these muscles that can be used as a landmark for anesthetic injections.[6] Addition of anesthesia to this area in combination with the sciatic block will theoretically block the entire foot. Multiple

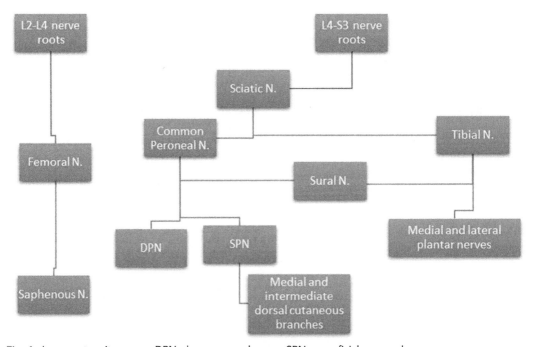

Fig. 1. Lower extremity nerves. DPN, deep peroneal nerve; SPN, superficial peroneal nerve.

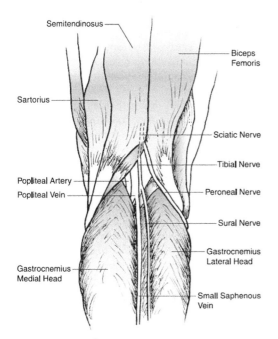

Fig. 2. Popliteal fossa.

variations have been reported for the saphenous nerve block, with data to support using trans-sartorial or subsartorial approaches. As the saphenous nerve courses distally to a level approximately 3 cm proximal to the medial malleolus, it divides into anterior and posterior branches, which each further ramify in the medial foot and ankle.[12,13] An accurate saphenous nerve block at the ankle level generally involves injecting just anterior and proximal to the medial malleolus (Fig. 3).

Ultrasound Versus Nerve Stimulator for Nerve Localization

Nerve blocks may be more safely performed by identifying the nerve before the injection (Fig. 4 and Table 1). Ultrasound guidance has replaced nerve stimulation as the preferred technique for nerve localization for peripheral nerve blocks.[17–20] A meta-analysis of 23 randomized controlled trials (RCTs) by Munirama and Mcleod[19] showed localization via ultrasound significantly reduced patient-reported procedural pain. Findings also included a decreased amount of anesthetic used and decreased inadvertent vascular punctures with the use of ultrasound. No difference in neurologic side effects was found between the 2 groups. Cao performed a separate meta-analysis of 10 RCTs comparing ultrasound versus nerve stimulation for nerve localization and found higher success and less vascular injuries with ultrasound guidance.[20] There were no significant differences on overall block success rate or procedure time.[19] A more recent report by Gelfand and

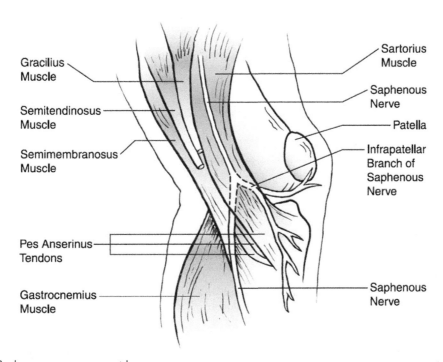

Fig. 3. Saphenous nerve course at knee.

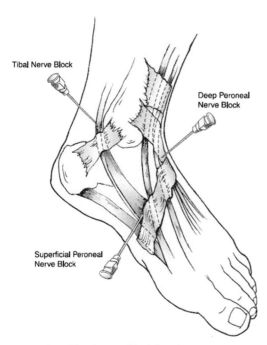

Tibal Nerve Block

Deep Peroneal
Nerve Block

Superficial Peroneal
Nerve Block

Fig. 4. Distal local nerve block locations.

colleagues[18] reviewed 16 RCTs and found ultrasound guidance was superior in overall block success compared with nerve stimulation in brachial plexus and popliteal sciatic blocks. Although the use of ultrasound is very operator-dependent, multiple studies report the use of ultrasound leads to better accuracy and clinical results when compared with nerve stimulation techniques.

Single-shot Versus Continuous Infusion

Reducing postoperative pain can be accomplished by a single injection or a continuous infusion via an indwelling catheter nerve block. The indwelling catheter necessary for a continuous nerve block may carry a small risk of infectious colonization[21] but provides longer term pain relief. Bingham and colleagues[7] reviewed 21 studies and found continuous blocks provided statistically significant better pain control on the first 3 postoperative days. In addition, continuous blocks were associated with fewer opioids, less nausea, and higher patient-satisfaction scores. Ding and colleagues[8] reported that subjects discharged with a continuous infusion nerve pump (Halyard; Irvine, CA, USA) had significantly lower pain scores and narcotic use at 2 and 12 weeks postoperatively compared with subjects who had a single-injection sciatic block after ankle fracture surgery. Another study on a subset of subjects undergoing surgical fixation of calcaneus fractures with postoperative continuous nerve blocks reported adequate pain control and postoperative day 1 discharge, with 63% lower total incurred costs.[5] Although indwelling catheters seem to provide increased duration of pain relief, many studies show effective pain control with single-shot blocks. Grosser and colleagues[22] looked at 25 consecutive subjects with preoperative popliteal blocks and found zero reported pain the in postanesthesia care unit. The average block duration was 14 hours and

Table 1 Lower extremity nerves		
	Distally	**Proximally**
Sural	Between Achilles and peroneal tendons; coursing with lesser saphenous vein	Posterior calf between 2 heads of gastrocnemius; coursing with lesser saphenous vein
Tibial	Posterior to medial malleolus, posterior to posterior tibial artery; between FDL and FHL	Between FDL and FHL in mid-tibia
Deep Peroneal Nerve	Between EHL and EDL, coursing with anterior tibial artery	On the IOM in anterior compartment of leg
Superficial Peroneal Nerve	Splits into dorsal and intermediate dorsal branches at the ankle	On the surface of peroneus brevis at midfibula in lateral compartment
Saphenous	Courses with saphenous vein and ramifies into anterior and posterior branches just proximal to medial malleolus. Effectively blocked slightly proximal and anterior to medial malleolus	Travels distally deep to pes tendons into subcutaneous tissue with the saphenous vein; gives off infrapatellar branch

Abbreviations: EDL, extensor digitorum longus; EHL, extensor hallucis longus; FDL, flexor digitorum longue; FHL, flexor hallucis longus; IOM, interosseous membrane.

subject satisfaction at 1 week was 4.8 out of 5. Elliot and colleagues[23] compared continuous versus single-shot blocks after hindfoot surgery and found the visual analog scale ranged from 1.1 to 3.6 in all subjects. The single-shot group did have statistically higher pain scores compared with the continuous group, but overall VAS scores were still low and likely not clinically significant. Single-shot blocks are also faster to perform and eliminate the need for a continuous pump. Ding and colleagues8 found 7 of 23 subjects in the continuous group had some degree of pump malfunction and 1 accidental catheter removal. Overall, the literature shows both options provide effective analgesia with each having its own benefits.

POSTOPERATIVE CARE AND REMOVAL

Although, in some surgical applications, peripheral nerve blocks may allow for more immediate rehabilitation, in foot and ankle surgery, nerve blocks must be used carefully because they may be associated with balance issues and falls.[24] Many foot and ankle procedures are followed by a postoperative regimen of nonweightbearing and limb elevation to minimize soft tissue swelling and promote healing. This postoperative protocol is also beneficial when nerve blocks are used because they eliminate the need for weightbearing on the insensate foot, which minimizes the effects of an insensate foot on balance and gait (Box 1).

AUTHORS' PREFERENCES

Patients undergoing foot and ankle surgery, whether elective or secondary to trauma, nearly always receive peripheral nerve blocks postoperatively. Before surgery, the anesthesiologist obtains consent and the details of the block are determined based on input from the patient and the surgeon. Concerns for compartment syndrome, whether from the injury sustained or procedure to be performed, are specific reasons that the surgeon may opt for not placing a nerve block (eg, acute tibial shaft fracture treated with intramedullary nailing). Procedures are generally conducted with limited gas or total intravenous anesthesia. A thigh tourniquet is frequently used. Injection of peri-incisional local anesthetic is generally withheld if the patient is to receive a continuous peripheral nerve block postoperatively. Once the skin is closed, a sterile dressing is applied to the surgical site, and a splint or walking boot is applied. The patient is

transferred to the postoperative holding unit where a member of the anesthesia team uses ultrasound to place the nerve block while the patient is still sedated from residual surgical anesthesia (Fig. 5).

Procedure details

- Supine position with the calf elevated on BoneFoam (Bone Foam, Inc, Corcoran, MN, USA)
- Prepped and draped in sterile fashion
- Ultrasound guidance to place a 30 cc ropivacaine bolus before catheter placement
- Catheter is placed and flushed, adhesive sterile dressings are applied, and the blocks are connected to the On-Q infusion pump (Halyard Health, Irvine, CA, USA)
- Home instruction sheet provided to the patient with a detailed care plan, including an on-call anesthesia nurse practitioner telephone number to call with any questions involving the nerve block and its removal (see Box 1).

Postoperative patients admitted to the hospital for 23-hour observation or inpatient stays are rounded on by an anesthesia staff member daily to insure block efficacy. If ineffective, the options include a bolus dose through the catheter, removal of catheter, or implantation of a new catheter.

There is ample time preoperatively for informed consent and patient education about the block by the anesthesia staff and, often, this has been discussed with the patient in their preoperative visit with the surgeon. In other settings it may be beneficial to have a designated anesthesia room to perform blocks preoperatively or postoperatively. There is no clear answer in the literature about which setting is most efficient, but it likely depends on each institution's resources. Brooks and colleagues[25] did show that consent and patient education by the anesthesia team the day before surgery led to 15% decrease in surgical case delays, as well as a 10% increase in the number of blocks used.

COMPLICATIONS
Neuropathic Symptoms
Neuropathic symptoms are the most commonly reported complications for nerve blocks.[9,26,27] Although most investigators report an incidence of less than 1% at final follow-up, some studies report a rate of residual symptoms approaching 25% at up to 6 months after

---

Box 1
Care instructions for the patient

Medication and infusion rate

- You will not see a change in the pump size for approximately 24 hours.
- When you notice pain and the sensation returning, you should take some of the pain medication you have been prescribed as directed.

For the patient with lower extremity peripheral nerve catheter

- Practice weightbearing as instructed, but you must use a walker or crutches at all times.

Notify nurse practitioner if the following occur:

- Inadequate pain control after using bolus button and taking oral pain medications
- Temperature greater than 101°F for 8 hours
- Increase in extremity numbness or weakness or trouble breathing
- Fluid will leak around the catheter: this is normal and does not mean it is not working. You may place a dressing at the catheter site, on top of the clear sterile bandage. The fluid may be clear or pink in color.

Stop infusion by clamping the tubing if you experience the following symptoms:

- Skin rash or hives, mouth or tongue numbness or tingling, ringing in the ears, blurred vision.

Information for infusion device daily use

- The medication reservoir should be protected from sunlight and heat.
- Do not shower, though you may sponge bathe. Do not immerse pump or catheter in water
- Do not inject anything into the catheter or tubing; this may result in severe limb injury or loss
- If at any point the dressing breaks down and the catheter becomes exposed to air, remove the catheter.

End of infusion

- You will have the infusion device system at home for 2 to 3 days.
- Stop the infusion when the device is empty (it will appear flat).
- Take prescribed oral medications as directed when the infusion system is ending.

To remove catheter

- Wash hands
- Turn infusion off by clamping the tubing and leave it clamped for 2 hours
- Remove dressing
- Slowly remove the catheter (it should come out easily with a gentle tug)
- After removing catheter, apply pressure with gauze for 5 minutes
- Examine catheter for a blue, black, or silver metal colored tip at the end
- If the tip is not there, or there is excessive pain when pulling the catheter, call the nurse practitioner
- Apply adhesive bandage as needed, inspect site for bleeding or swelling.

---

surgery.[28] In Anderson and colleagues'[29] study of 1014 subjects, 5% had postoperative neuropathic symptoms and .7% had residual symptoms at the final follow-up. The investigators found no significant different with use of nerve stimulation, steroid use, diabetes, or tourniquet location. Gartke and colleagues[28] reported a much higher incidence of neuropathic symptoms after popliteal blocks, with smokers experiencing a significantly increased risk for residual neuropathic symptoms. Overall, most investigators report a relatively low incidence of postprocedure neuropathic symptoms that can be attributed to nerve blocks. However, this should remain a part of the informed consent process.

Infection

Indwelling peripheral nerve catheters after foot and ankle surgery may pose a slight risk as a

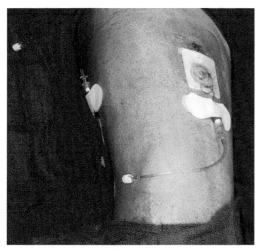

Fig. 5. (*Left*) Continuous sciatic popliteal nerve block. (*Right*) Continuous saphenous nerve block (before infusion bulbs).

possible source of infection. Capdevila and colleagues[21] reported up to a 57% colonization rate with up to 3% subsequent infection in their review of 1,416 subjects undergoing orthopedic procedures. Independent risk factors for infection included catheter use greater than 48 hours, lack of prophylactic antibiotics, intensive care unit (ICU) status, and axillary or femoral catheters as opposed to other locations. ICU status and catheter use greater than 48 hours had the highest odds ratio for infection and local inflammation, at 5.07 and 4.61, respectively. The most common microorganism found when obtaining cultures was *Staphylococcus*. Another evaluation 2,285 peripheral nerve catheters reported a 3.2% infection rate with .9% requiring surgical intervention. The investigators found that anterior sciatic catheters were at a significantly lower risk of infection when compared with other upper and lower extremity catheters.[30] The largest

review of peripheral nerve catheter-associated infections found infection rates of 0% to 3.2%.[21] Although only a small percentage of the catheters being placed develop infection, there are exceedingly more rare reports of necrotizing fasciitis as a complication.[31]

Compartment Syndrome

Multiple studies have looked at the efficacy of indwelling peripheral nerve blocks after fracture treatment in the lower extremity.[2,5,8,32,33] Although the anesthesia blunts early postoperative pain, it also limits the clinicians' capacity for an accurate physical examination by leaving the foot commonly insensate and without motor function. Although extremely rare, compartment syndrome of the foot is a devastating consequence that may be initially masked by a peripheral nerve block. Cometa and colleagues[34] presented the case of a 15-year-old patient who underwent tibial and femoral osteotomies with external fixation to correct Blount deformity with postoperative femoral and sciatic nerve indwelling catheters. Despite a peripheral block and oral medications, the patient still experienced severe pain and had a physical examination consistent with compartment syndrome on postoperative day 2. Other investigators note the importance of pain in diagnosing compartment syndrome of the leg after tibial shaft fractures, where pain appears to be the predominant symptom.[35] Davis and colleagues[36] reported that some form of regional anesthesia was reported as being used in 26% to 34% of tibial fractures. Of those that were diagnosed with a compartment syndrome, a spinal epidural was used in 88%.

A case report by Noorpuri and colleagues[37] documents a foot compartment syndrome after revision arthroplasties of the forefoot. Local 1-time blocks were administered to the

Table 2
Signs of anesthetic toxicity

System	Early Signs	At Increased Concentrations
Neurologic	Perioral tingling, light-headedness, dizziness, blurred vison, tinnitus	Tremor, muscle twitching; generalized tonic-clonic seizures; CNS depression, coma
Cardiac	Hypertension, tachycardia	Ventricular arrhythmias, conduction delays; profound contractile dysfunction with cardiovascular collapse
Treatment	• ACLS protocol to secure airway, suppress arrhythmias and sustain blood pressure • Intralipid administration • Seizure control	

Abbreviations: ACLS, advanced cardiac life support; CNS, central nervous system.

forefoot for procedural anesthesia. The diagnosis was made approximately 12 hours later when pain was not relieved with elevation and oral pain medications. The patient's examination was consistent with compartment syndrome of the foot. Although rare, especially in the realm of elective foot and ankle surgeries, the surgeon must maintain a concern for compartment syndrome and understand peripheral nerve blocks may mask the earliest symptoms.

Local anesthetic systemic toxicity considerations include

- Incidence: 7.5 to 20 per 10,000 all nerve blocks performed[38]
- Patients with cardiac, renal, and hepatic impairment may need reduced amounts of anesthetic
- Elderly and pregnant patients may also need reduced dosing (Table 2).

SUMMARY

Peripheral nerve blocks have proven to be a safe addition to the multitude of modalities for perioperative pain control. Among the primary benefits, they allow for decreased narcotic use, earlier discharge, and decreased hospital cost for the patient. Patients should be counseled on the most common side effects of peripheral nerve blocks, which include local inflammation, infection, and the possibility of prolonged neuropathic symptoms.

REFERENCES

1. Singelyn FJ, Aye F, Gouverneur JM. Continuous popliteal sciatic nerve block: an original technique to provide postoperative analgesia after foot surgery. Anesth Analg 1997;84:383–6. Availble at: http://dx.doi.org/10.1097/00000539-199702000-00027.
2. Luiten WE, Schepers T, Luitse JS, et al. Comparison of continuous nerve block versus patient-controlled analgesia for postoperative pain and outcome after talar and calcaneal fractures. Foot Ankle Int 2014; 35(11):1116–21.
3. Capdevila X, Pirat P, Bringuier S, et al. Continuous peripheral nerve blocks in hospital wards after orthopedic surgery: a multicenter prospective analysis of the quality of postoperative analgesia and complications in 1,416 patients. Anesthesiology 2005;103(5):1035–45.
4. Pakzad H, Thevendran G, Penner MJ, et al. Factors associated with longer length of hospital stay after primary elective ankle surgery for end-stage ankle arthritis. J Bone Joint Surg Am 2014;96(1):32–9.
5. Hunt KJ, Higgins TF, Carlston CV, et al. Continuous peripheral nerve blockade as postoperative analgesia for open treatment of calcaneal fractures. J Orthop Trauma 2010;24(3):148–55.
6. Swenson J, Davis JJ. Anesthesia. In: Coughlin MJ, Saltzman CL, Mann RA, editors. Mann's surgery of the foot and ankle. 9th edition. Saunders: Elsevier; 2014. p. 135–48.
7. Bingham A, Fu R, Horn JL, et al. Continuous peripheral nerve block compared with single-injection peripheral nerve block : a systematic review and meta-analysis of randomized controlled trials. Reg Anesth Pain Med 2012;37(6):583–94.
8. Ding DY, Manoli A 3rd, Galos DK, et al. Continuous popliteal sciatic nerve block versus single injection nerve block for ankle fracture surgery: a prospective randomized comparative trial. J Orthop Trauma 2015;29(9):393–8.
9. Hajek V. Neuropathic complications after 157 procedures of continuous popliteal nerve block for hallux valgus surgery. A retrospective study. Orthop Traumatol Surg Res 2012;98(3):327–33.
10. Grebing BR, Coughlin MJ. Evaluation of the Esmark bandage as a tourniquet for forefoot surgery. Foot Ankle Int 2004;26(6):397–405.
11. Michelson J, Perry M. Clinical safety and efficacy of calf tourniquets. Foot Ankle Int 1996;17(9):573–5.
12. Aszmann OC, Ebmer JM, Dellon AL. Cutaneous innervation of the medial ankle: an anatomic study of the saphenous, sural, and tibial nerves and their clinical significance. Foot Ankle Int 1998;19:753–6.
13. Mercer D, Morrell NT, Fitzpatrick J, et al. The course of the distal saphenous nerve: a cadaveric investigation and clinical implications. Iowa Orthop J 2011;31:231–5.
14. Marsland D, Dray A, Little NJ, et al. The saphenous nerve in foot and ankle surgery: its variable anatomy and relevance. Foot Ankle Surg 2013;19(2):76–9.
15. Benzon HT, Sharma S, Calimaran A. Comparison of the different approaches to saphenous nerve block. Anesthesiology 2005;102(3):633–8.
16. Mentzel M, Fleischmann W, Bauer G, et al. Ankle joint denervation. Part 1: Anatomy –the sensory innervation of the ankle joint. Foot Ankle Surg 1999;5:15–20.
17. Abrahams MS, Aziz MF, Fu RF, et al. Ultrasound guidance compared with electrical neurostimulation for peripheral nerve block: a systematic review and meta-analysis of randomized controlled trials. Br J Anaesth 2009;102:408–17.
18. Gelfand HJ, Ouanes JP, Lesley MR, et al. Analgesic efficacy of ultrasound-guided regional anesthesia: a meta-analysis. J Clin Anesth 2011;23:90–6.
19. Munirama S, Mcleod G. A systematic review and meta-analysis of ultrasound versus electrical

stimulation for peripheral nerve location and blockade. Anesthesia 2015;70:1084–91.

20. Cao X, Zhao X, Xu J, et al. Ultrasound-guided technology versus neurostimulation for sciatic nerver block: a meta-analysis. Int J Clin Exp Med 2015; 8(1):273–80.

21. Capdevila X, Bringuier S, Borgeat A. Infectious risk of continuous peripheral nerve blocks. Anesthesiology 2009;110:182–8.

22. Grosser D, Herr M, Claridge R. Preoperative lateral popliteal nerve block for intraoperative and postoperative pain control in elective foot and ankle surgery: a prospective analysis. Foot Ankle Int 2005;28(12):1271–5.

23. Elliot R, Pearce C, Seifert C, et al. Preoperative lateral popliteal nerve block for intraoperative and postoperative pain control in elective foot and ankle surgery: a prospective analysis. Foot Ankle Int 2010;28(12):1043–7.

24. Xing JG, Abdallah FW, Brull R, et al. Preoperative femoral nerve block for hip arthroscopy: a randomized, triple-masked controlled trial. Am J Sports Med 2015;43(11):2680–7.

25. Brooks B, Barman J, Ponce B, et al. An electronic surgical order, undertaking patient education, and obtaining informed consent for regional analgesia before the day of surgery reduce block-related delays. Local Reg Anesth 2016;9:59–64.

26. Barrington MJ, Snyder GL. Neurologic complications of regional anesthesia. Curr Opin Anaesthesiol 2011;24:554–60.

27. Brull R, McCartney CJ, Chan VW, et al. Neurological complications after regional anesthesia: contemporary estimates of risk. Anesth Analg 2007;104:965–74.

28. Gartke K, Portner O, Taljaard M. Neuropathic symptoms following continuous popliteal block after foot and ankle surgery. Foot Ankle Int 2012;33: 267–74.

29. Anderson JG, Bohay DR, Maskill JD, et al. Complications after popliteal block for foot and ankle surgery. Foot Ankle Int 2015;36(10):1138–43.

30. Neuburger M, Büttner J, Blumenthal S, et al. Inflammation and infection complications of 2285 perineural catheters: a prospective study. Acta Anaesthesiol Scand 2007;51:108–14.

31. Dott D, Canlas C, Sobey C, et al. Necrotizing fasciitis as a complication of a continuous sciatic nerve catheter using the lateral popliteal approach. Reg Anesth Pain Med 2016;41(6):728–30.

32. Goldstein RY, Montero N, Jain SK, et al. Efficacy of popliteal block in postoperative pain control after ankle fracture fixation: a prospective randomized study. J Orthop Trauma 2012;26(10):557–61.

33. Cooper J, Benirschke S, Sangeorzan B, et al. Sciatic nerve blockade improves early postoperative analgesia after open repair of calcaneus fractures. J Orthop Trauma 2004;18(4):197–201.

34. Cometa MA, Esch AT, Boezaart AP, et al. Did continuous femoral and sciatic nerve block obscure the diagnosis or delay the treatment of acute lower leg compartment syndrome? A case report. Pain Med 2011;12:823–8.

35. Munk-Anderson H, Laustrup TK. Compartment syndrome diagnosed in due time by breakthrough pain despite continuous peripheral nerve block. Acta Anaesthesiol Scand 2013;57:1328–30.

36. Davis ET, Harris A, Keene D, et al. The use of regional anaesthesia in patients at risk of acute compartment syndrome. Injury 2006;37: 128–33.

37. Noorpuri BS, Shahane SA, Getty CJ, et al. Acute compartment syndrome following revisional arthroplasty of the forefoot: the dangers of ankle-block. Foot Ankle Int 2000;21(8):680–2.

38. Dillane D. Local anesthetic systemic toxicity. Can J Anaesth 2010;57:368–80.

UNITED STATES POSTAL SERVICE®

Statement of Ownership, Management, and Circulation (All Periodicals Publications Except Requester Publications)

1. Publication Title	2. Publication Number	3. Filing Date
ORTHOPEDIC CLINICS OF NORTH AMERICA	950 – 920	9/18/2017

4. Issue Frequency	5. Number of Issues Published Annually	6. Annual Subscription Price
JAN, APR, JUL, OCT	4	$319.00

7. Complete Mailing Address of Known Office of Publication (Not printer) (Street, city, county, state, and ZIP+4®)

ELSEVIER INC.
230 Park Avenue, Suite 800
New York, NY 10169

Contact Person
STEPHEN R. BUSHING

Telephone (Include area code)
215-239-3688

8. Complete Mailing Address of Headquarters or General Business Office of Publisher (Not printer)

ELSEVIER INC.
230 Park Avenue, Suite 800
New York, NY 10169

9. Full Names and Complete Mailing Addresses of Publisher, Editor, and Managing Editor (Do not leave blank)

Publisher (Name and complete mailing address)

ADRIANNE BRIGIDO, ELSEVIER INC.
1600 JOHN F KENNEDY BLVD. SUITE 1800
PHILADELPHIA, PA 19103-2899

Editor (Name and complete mailing address)

LAUREN BOYLE, ELSEVIER INC.
1600 JOHN F KENNEDY BLVD. SUITE 1800
PHILADELPHIA, PA 19103-2899

Managing Editor (Name and complete mailing address)

PATRICK MANLEY, ELSEVIER INC.
1600 JOHN F KENNEDY BLVD. SUITE 1800
PHILADELPHIA, PA 19103-2899

10. Owner (Do not leave blank. If the publication is owned by a corporation, give the name and address of the corporation immediately followed by the names and addresses of all stockholders owning or holding 1 percent or more of the total amount of stock. If not owned by a corporation, give the names and addresses of the individual owners. If owned by a partnership or other unincorporated firm, give its name and address as well as those of each individual owner. If the publication is published by a nonprofit organization, give its name and address.)

Full Name	Complete Mailing Address
WHOLLY OWNED SUBSIDIARY OF REED/ELSEVIER US HOLDINGS	1600 JOHN F KENNEDY BLVD. SUITE 1800 PHILADELPHIA, PA 19103-2899

11. Known Bondholders, Mortgagees, and Other Security Holders Owning or Holding 1 Percent or More of Total Amount of Bonds, Mortgages, or Other Securities. If none, check box ► ☐ None

Full Name	Complete Mailing Address
N/A	

12. Tax Status (For completion by nonprofit organizations authorized to mail at nonprofit rates) (Check one)
The purpose, function, and nonprofit status of this organization and the exempt status for federal income tax purposes:
☒ Has Not Changed During Preceding 12 Months
☐ Has Changed During Preceding 12 Months (Publisher must submit explanation of change with this statement)

PS Form 3526, July 2014 [Page 1 of 4 (see instructions page 4)] PSN: 7530-01-000-9931 PRIVACY NOTICE: See our privacy policy on www.usps.com.

---

13. Publication Title	14. Issue Date for Circulation Data Below
ORTHOPEDIC CLINICS OF NORTH AMERICA	JULY 2017

15. Extent and Nature of Circulation			Average No. Copies Each Issue During Preceding 12 Months	No. Copies of Single Issue Published Nearest to Filing Date
a. Total Number of Copies (Net press run)			337	405
b. Paid Circulation (By Mail and Outside the Mail)	(1)	Mailed Outside-County Paid Subscriptions Stated on PS Form 3541 (include paid distribution above nominal rate, advertiser's proof copies, and exchange copies)	91	130
	(2)	Mailed In-County Paid Subscriptions Stated on PS Form 3541 (include paid distribution above nominal rate, advertiser's proof copies, and exchange copies)	0	0
	(3)	Paid Distribution Outside the Mails Including Sales Through Dealers and Carriers, Street Vendors, Counter Sales, and Other Paid Distribution Outside USPS®	110	192
	(4)	Paid Distribution by Other Classes of Mail Through the USPS (e.g. First-Class Mail®)	0	0
c. Total Paid Distribution (Sum of 15b (1), (2), (3), and (4))		►	201	322
d. Free or Nominal Rate Distribution (By Mail and Outside the Mail)	(1)	Free or Nominal Rate Outside-County Copies included on PS Form 3541	60	83
	(2)	Free or Nominal Rate In-County Copies Included on PS Form 3541	0	0
	(3)	Free or Nominal Rate Copies Mailed at Other Classes Through the USPS (e.g. First-Class Mail)	0	0
	(4)	Free or Nominal Rate Distribution Outside the Mail (Carriers or other means)	0	0
e. Total Free or Nominal Rate Distribution (Sum of 15d (1), (2), (3) and (4))		►	60	83
f. Total Distribution (Sum of 15c and 15e)		►	261	405
g. Copies not Distributed (See Instructions to Publishers #4 (page #3))		►	76	0
h. Total (Sum of 15f and g)		►	337	405
i. Percent Paid (15c divided by 15f times 100)		►	77.01%	79.51%

* If you are claiming electronic copies, go to line 16 on page 3. If you are not claiming electronic copies, skip to line 17 on page 3.

16. Electronic Copy Circulation		Average No. Copies Each Issue During Preceding 12 Months	No. Copies of Single Issue Published Nearest to Filing Date
a. Paid Electronic Copies	►	0	0
b. Total Paid Print Copies (Line 15c) + Paid Electronic Copies (Line 16a)	►	201	322
c. Total Print Distribution (Line 15f) + Paid Electronic Copies (Line 16a)	►	261	405
d. Percent Paid (Both Print & Electronic Copies) (16b divided by 16c × 100)	►	77.01%	79.51%

☒ I certify that 50% of all my distributed copies (electronic and print) are paid above a nominal price.

17. Publication of Statement of Ownership

☒ If the publication is a general publication, publication of this statement is required. Will be printed in the OCTOBER 2017 issue of this publication.   ☐ Publication not required.

18. Signature and Title of Editor, Publisher, Business Manager or Owner		Date
Stephen R. Bushing		9/18/2017

STEPHEN R. BUSHING - INVENTORY DISTRIBUTION CONTROL MANAGER

I certify that all information furnished on this form is true and complete. I understand that anyone who furnishes false or misleading information on this form or who omits material or information requested on the form may be subject to criminal sanctions (including fines and imprisonment) and/or civil sanctions (including civil penalties).

PS Form 3526, July 2014 (Page 3 of 4) PRIVACY NOTICE: See our privacy policy on www.usps.com

Printed and bound by CPI Group (UK) Ltd, Croydon, CR0 4YY

08/05/2025

01864703-0016